Healthcare Systems and Health Informatics

Innovations in Health Informatics and Healthcare: Using Artificial Intelligence and Smart Computing

Series Editors

Rashmi Agrawal, Manav Rachna International Institute of Research and Studies and *Mamta Mittal, G.B. Pant Government Engineering College*

The aim of this series is to publish reference books and handbooks that will provide conceptual and advanced reference material centered around Health Informatics and Healthcare using AI and Smart Computing. There are numerous fields within the healthcare sector where these technologies are applicable including successful ways of handling patients during a pandemic time. Large volumes of data, data analysis, smart computing devices like IoT for sensing health data have drastically changed the way the healthcare sector functions. The scope of the book series is to report the latest advances and developments in the field of Health Informatics with the use of the latest technologies. Each book will describe in detail the use of AI, Smart Computing, Evolutionary Computing, Deep Learning, and Data Analysis in the field of Health Informatics and the books will include real-life problems that focus on the Healthcare System.

Intelligent Computing Applications for COVID-19
Predictions, Diagnosis, and Prevention
Edited by Tanzila Saba and Amjad Rehman

Blockchain for Healthcare Systems
Challenges, Privacy, and Securing of Data
Edited by Shiekh Mohammad Idrees, Paural Agarwal, and M. Afshar Alam

Healthcare Systems and Health Informatics
Using Internet of Things
Edited by Pawan Singh Mehra, Lalit Mohan Goyal, Arvind Dagur, and Anshu Kumar Dwivedi

For more information on this series, please visit: https://www.routledge.com/ Innovations-in-Health-Informatics-and-Healthcare-Using-Artificial-Intelligence-and-Smart-Computing/book-series/CRCIHIHUAISM

Healthcare Systems and Health Informatics

Using Internet of Things

Edited by
Pawan Singh Mehra, Lalit Mohan Goyal, Arvind Dagur, and
Anshu Kumar Dwivedi

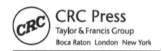

CRC Press
Taylor & Francis Group
Boca Raton London New York

CRC Press is an imprint of the
Taylor & Francis Group, an **informa** business

First edition published 2022
by CRC Press
6000 Broken Sound Parkway NW, Suite 300, Boca Raton, FL 33487-2742

and by CRC Press
4 Park Square, Milton Park, Abingdon, Oxon, OX14 4RN

Library of Congress Cataloging-in-Publication Data
Names: Mehra, Pawan Singh, editor. | Goyal, Lalit Mohan, editor. |
Dagur, Arvind, editor. | Dwivedi, Anshu Kumar, editor.
Title: Healthcare systems and health informatics : using internet of
things / edited by Pawan Singh Mehra, Lalit Mohan Goyal,
Arvind Dagur, and Anshu Kumar Dwivedi.
Description: First edition. | Boca Raton : CRC Press, 2022. |
Series: Innovations in health informatics and healthcare: using
artificial intelligence and smart computing |
Includes bibliographical references and index.
Identifiers: LCCN 2021043550 (print) | LCCN 2021043551 (ebook) |
ISBN 9780367703943 (hardback) | ISBN 9780367703950 (paperback) |
ISBN 9781003146087 (ebook)
Subjects: LCSH: Medical informatics. | Medical care.
Classification: LCC R858 .H436 2022 (print) |
LCC R858 (ebook) | DDC 610.285–dc23/eng/20211209
LC record available at https://lccn.loc.gov/2021043550
LC ebook record available at https://lccn.loc.gov/2021043551

ISBN: 978-0-367-70394-3 (hbk)
ISBN: 978-0-367-70395-0 (pbk)
ISBN: 978-1-003-14608-7 (ebk)

DOI: 10.1201/9781003146087

Typeset in Times
by Newgen Publishing UK

Contents

UNIT 1 Introduction to IoT-Based Healthcare Devices

UNIT 2 IoT-Based Systems for Healthcare Sector: AI and Smart Computing

UNIT 3 IoT-Based Systems for Healthcare Industries: Opportunities and Challenges

UNIT 4 Security and Privacy in IoT-Based Systems for Healthcare Sector

Preface

Kevin Ashton coined the term Internet of Things (IoT) in the year 1999. IOT can impact our daily lives by providing any service to anyone at any point in time. One of the potential applications of IoT can be health informatics and healthcare. This book provides a comprehensive description of the essential aspects of IoT and health from beginner to advanced level perspectives. It describes the fundamentals of IoT and healthcare wherein discussions are carried out for system architecture, protocols, wearable devices, interoperability, and different applications of IoT in healthcare. The impact of artificial intelligence and smart computing is provided for depicting the enhancement of existing systems. Challenges and opportunities for the healthcare industry are discussed for maximal societal benefits. With more and more advancement and daily usage of IoT based healthcare devices, improvements and enhancements for information security and security devices are required by adopting a security-focused approach with increased transparency to the user. This book is compiled to address maximal issues in IoT-based healthcare with some existing improved solutions.

Editors

Pawan Singh Mehra is an Assistant Professor at Delhi Technological University, New Delhi, India. He earned a PhD in computer engineering at Jamia Millia Islamia and MTech (Hons) in computer science and engineering at the Center for Development of Advanced Computing (CDAC). He earned a BE at RJIT, Gwalior. He has approximately ten years of teaching and research experience. He has authored more than 25 publications in international conferences and journals indexed in SCI, Scopus, ESCI, and Web of Science. His research interests include wireless sensor network, internet of things, image processing, cryptography, and network security and blockchain.

Lalit Mohan Goyal earned a PhD at Jamia Millia Islamia, New Delhi in computer engineering, an MTech (Hons) in information technology at Guru Gobind Singh Indraprastha University, New Delhi, and a BTech (Hons) in computer engineering at Kurukshetra University, Kurukshetra. He has 16 years of teaching experience in the theory of computation, parallel and random algorithms, distributed data mining, and cloud computing. He has completed a project sponsored by the Indian Council of Medical Research, Delhi. He has published many research papers in SCI-indexed and Scopus-indexed journals and conferences. Two patents filed by him are also now published online. He is reviewer of many reputed journals and conferences. He has given many invited talks in FDP and conferences. Presently, he a faculty member in the Department of Computer Engineering at J.C. Bose University of Science and Technology, YMCA Faridabad.

Arvind Dagur is working as a Professor in Department of Computer Science and Engineering, Galgotias University, India. He completed his Ph.D. (Computer Engineering) from Jamia Millia Islamia, New Delhi, India, M. Tech. (Computer Science and Engineering) from MNNIT, Allahabad, India, and B.Tech. (CSE) from UPTU. He has more than 16 Years of experience in various reputed colleges such as KIET Group, AKGEC, ABESIT, and Galgotias College of Engineering and Technology. He has published more than 30 research papers in reputed international Journals / Conferences. He also published 5 book chapters in Springer Book series such as LNCS, AICS Series, and LNICST. His area of research is real time scheduling, cloud computing and IoT.

Anshu Kumar Dwivedi is currently working as Associate Professor and Head in department of Computer Science and Engineering at Buddha Institute of Technology, Gorakhpur, India. He received his Ph.D. degree in Computer Science & Engineering from Madan Mohan Malaviya University of Technology, Gorakhpur, and M.Tech (HONS) degree in Computer Engineering from YMCA University of Science and Technology, Faridabad, India. He completed Bachelor of Technology from UPTU, Lucknow, India. He has also cleared GATE 2010, 2011, 2018 and got MHRD scholarship. His research interests include wireless sensor network, image processing, Artificial intelligence, and Data Science. He has authored a book theory of automata and formal language and other two are in progress. He has published several research articles in leading SCI Index International Journals from IEEE, Elsevier, Springer, John Wiley, etc. He is reviewer of Scopus/SCI Indexed International Journals.

Contributors

Reshu Agarwal
Amity Institute of Information
  Technology
Amity University
Noida, Uttar Pradesh, India

Shruti Agarwal
Department of Computer Science and
  Engineering
Meerut Institute of Engineering and
  Technology
Meerut, Uttar Pradesh, India

Safaa N. Saud Al-Humairi
Faculty of Information Sciences and
  Engineering
Management and Science University
Shah Alam, Selangor, Malaysia

Salah Al-Zubaidi
Department of Automated
  Manufacturing Engineering
Al-Khwarizmi College of
  Engineering
University of Baghdad
Baghdad, Iraq

Sanyam Arora
Department of Computer Science and
  Engineering
Meerut Institute of Engineering and
  Technology
Meerut, Uttar Pradesh, India

Siti Humairah Kamarul Bahrain
Department of Engineering and
  Technology
Faculty of Information Sciences and
  Engineering
Management and Science University
Shah Alam, Selangor, Malaysia

Ritin Behl
Department of Information
  Technology
ABES Engineering College
Ghaziabad, Uttar Pradesh, India

Debanjan Chatterjee
Department of Natural Products
National Institute of Pharmaceutical
  Education and Research
Gandhinagar, Gujarat, India

Luv Dhamija
Department of Computer Science and
  Engineering
ABES Engineering College
Ghaziabad, Uttar Pradesh, India

Brainvendra Widi Dionova
Department of Electrical
  Engineering
Jakarta Global University
Depok, West Java, Indonesia

Asmita Dixit
Jaypee Institute of Information
  Technology
Noida, Uttar Pradesh, India

Karan Gupta
Department of Information
  Technology
ABES Engineering College
Ghaziabad, Uttar Pradesh, India

Asif Iqbal Hajamydeen
Faculty of Information Sciences and
  Engineering
Management and Science
  University
Shah Alam, Selangor, Malaysia

Wahida Handouzi
LAT Laboratory
Tlemcen University
Tlemcen, Algeria

Ashwini R. Hirekodi
Osteos India Pvt. Ltd.
Belagavi, Karnataka, India

Kaouter Karboub
FRDISI and ENSEM
Hassan II University
Casablanca, Morocco

Kuldeep Singh Kaswan
School of Computing Science and
    Technology
Galgotias University
Greater Noida, Uttar Pradesh, India

Inderpreet Kaur
Computer Science and Engineering
Galgotias College of Engineering and
    Technology
Greater Noida, Uttar Pradesh, India

Mukul Kumar
G.L. Bajaj Institute of Technology and
    Management
Greater Noida, Uttar Pradesh, India

Naresh Kumar
School of Computing Science and
    Technology
Galgotias University
Greater Noida, Uttar Pradesh, India

Sanjay Kumar
Information Technology
Galgotias College of Engineering and
    Technology
Greater Noida, Uttar Pradesh, India

Vimal Kumar
Department of Computer Science and
    Engineering
Meerut Institute of Engineering and
    Technology
Meerut, Uttar Pradesh, India

Chandrajit M.
Maharaja Research Foundation
Maharaja Institute of
    Technology Mysore
Mandya, Karnataka, India

Anil B. Malali
Department of Commerce and
    Management
Acharya Institute of Graduate Studies
Bengaluru, Karnataka, India

Chandan Kumar Malik
Department of Pharmaceutical
    Technology
Jadavpur University
Kolkata, West Bengal, India

Gourav Mitawa
Sobhasaria Group of Institutions
Sikar, Rajasthan, India

M.N. Mohammed
Department of Engineering and
    Technology
Faculty of Information Sciences and
    Engineering
Management and Science University
Shah Alam, Selangor, Malaysia

Sumathy Mohan
Department of Commerce
Bharathiyar University
Coimbatore, Tamil Nadu, India

Manohar N.
Department of Computer Science
Amrita School of Arts and Science,
    Mysuru Campus
Mysore, Karnataka, India

Shobha Rani N.
Department of Computer Science
Amrita School of Arts and Science,
    Mysuru Campus
Bhogadi, Karnataka, India

Aparajita Nanda
Jaypee Institute of Information
    Technology
Noida, Uttar Pradesh, India

Jin Yong Park
Konkuk School of Business
Konkuk University
Gwangjin-gu, Seoul, South Korea

Bhagyashri Pandurangi R.
Department of Electronics and
  Communication Engineering
KLS Gogte Institute of Technology
Belagavi, Karnataka, India

Bipin Kumar Rai
IT Department
ABES Institute of Technology
Ghaziabad, Uttar Pradesh, India

Husniza Razalli
Faculty of Information Sciences and
  Engineering
Management and Science
  University
Shah Alam, Selangor, Malaysia

Luv Sethi
Department of Computer Science and
  Engineering
Meerut Institute of Engineering and
  Technology
Meerut, Uttar Pradesh, India

Sanjeev Kumar Singh
Information Technology Department
Galgotias College of Engineering and
  Technology
Greater Noida, Uttar Pradesh, India

Gopalakrishnan Subramanian
Department of Commerce and
  Management
Acharya Institute of Graduate Studies
Bengaluru, Karnataka, India

Vasudev T.
Maharaja Research Foundation
Maharaja Institute of
  Technology Mysore
Mandya, Karnataka, India

Mohamed Tabaa
LPRI EMSI Casablanca
Casablanca, Morocco

Dhanabalan Thangam
Department of Commerce and
  Management
Acharya Institute of Graduate Studies
Bengaluru, Karnataka, India

Eddy Yusuf
Faculty of Pharmacy
Jakarta Global University
Depok, West Java, Indonesia

Unit 1

Introduction to IoT-Based Healthcare Devices

1 Internet of Things
A Smart Technology for Healthcare Industries

Dhanabalan Thangam, Anil B. Malali, and Gopalakrishnan Subramanian
Department of Commerce and Management
Acharya Institute of Graduate Studies

Sumathy Mohan
Department of Commerce
Bharathiyar University

Jin Yong Park
Konkuk School of Business
Konkuk University

CONTENTS

DOI: 10.1201/9781003146087-2

Technological advancements occupy almost all fields, especially in the field of healthcare. Lots of chronic diseases have threatened the present world due to various reasons. This results in a lot of developments in the healthcare field every year, technically and medicinally. Modern medical technologies provide better patient care and make the doctors' work easier than ever before. Moreover, wide research has been conducted on various information technologies (IT) related to integrating and promoting healthcare services. Very specifically, IT-enabled tools such as the Internet of Things (IoT), artificial intelligence (AI), big data analysis are contributing a lot in promoting the healthcare industry. Exceptionally the IoT has been enforced extensively to integrate the current healthcare industry resources for offering reliable, efficient, and agile medical services to aged patients and patients with continual illness. Besides, IoT has various utilisations in the medical field, such as safeguarding and monitoring patients and improving patients' care. Thus, IoT ensures enhanced care for patients by facilitating them to spend extra time with the medical practitioners.

On the other hand, IoT has its shortcomings, such as maintaining more medical instruments and collecting a vast amount of data that can be troublesome for hospital IT staff to supervise and manage. Furthermore, keeping patients' information secure is a big issue, especially when relocated between various instruments. With this backdrop, the present chapter has been prepared to sum up the relevance of IoT in the patient care sector and establish the recent trends and future course of action for potential research in this field.

1.1   INTRODUCTION

Human health has been at risk in recent years due to overpopulation, and it also leads to a lot of diseases. As a result, there is a need for superior healthcare technology, and it should have the capability to curtail these conditions as much as possible. At present, the healthcare industry is developing quickly with innovative technologies. There is a rising need for healthcare, caused by issues such as an increase in unceasing illnesses to the worldwide populace, limited hospitals, healthcare professionals, and various service providers, to provide very good healthcare services for getting better patient outcomes [1]. All such problems pave the way for utilising the latest tools like the IoT, artificial intelligence, machine learning, and data analytics. Amongst these, IoT has supported a lot of health-related service providers. In the Industry 4.0 era, applying IT enabled technologies for healthcare services has become well-liked after proposing various novel thoughts, like Smart earth and City [2]. Every business sector contributes a lot towards the growth and development of the economy of any country and makes a difference. However, the healthcare industry is habitually considered to be a very important sector. [3].

Meanwhile, it is also complicated, more so as it engages in providing accurate medical attention to the deprived at an exact time. The pre-Internet era would see an enormous process associated with every activity concerned with the healthcare process. Still, ever since technology took over, there has been a lot of transformation. One such enormous support from technology towards the development of the healthcare system is the influx of IoT into the health industry [4]. The materialisation of IoT makes the healthcare industry smarter, faster, and stronger than ever before. The IoT is facilitated to interconnect healthcare appliances like supervising healthcare systems, sensor technologies, and other pointing devices that can determine and retain real-time health-related data. The pointing devices collect and store health-related data on federal cloud storage systems or servers to analyse the healthcare data for taking a health-related decision and provide better treatment [5].

Moreover, the overall IoT's market share in the healthcare industry is projected to grow USD 188 billion by 2024, at a compound annual growth rate (CAGR) of 27.6% in the same period [6]. So the major players in this industry are endeavouring to grasp the benefits of this expansion and improve their results by investing more in such advanced technologies. According to the Medical Device Network report [7], by 2030 40% of IoT-related technologies would be utilised in the health and medical industry. As of today, IoT in the medical sector has around 22% of the entire IoT market. Internationally, about 60% of health-related institutions have already put into practice IoT outcomes. In the forthcoming years, it is expected that the number of users or patients and practitioners in the healthcare industry who will be using IoT-linked devices for monitoring health will rise to 44.4% each year [8]. The development potential of IoT in the global healthcare sector is discussed in Ray (2016) [9]. The role of IoT in the health sector contains much harm that comes with matters related to medicine all through history. However, the IoT and health sector can equally give better results.

1.2   REALISING THE ROLE OF IOT IN THE HEALTH SECTOR

The rising needs of the health sector have made innovation necessary for health-related services to render excellent health-related services. There are numerous gains that can be realised by using IoT in the health industry, such as facilitating the concurrent observation of the patients, offering a wide range of well-established tracks to gather patients' data, and checking the actions of hospitals, staff, and patients properly to meet the new needs, such as getting a superior consideration of the patient's health situation in a sequence of stages and multifaceted concern needs, focusing on a contemporary patient care approach and healthcare deliverance system design, clinical as well as a scientific data structure to supporting decisions, and an elegant continuing healthcare programme developed by an integrative panel [9]. IoT in the health industry is supportive at various places of the interaction between patients and health technology. The primary stage starts with the patients while making their call for booking appointments to the hospital or visiting the hospital directly in urgent situations [10]. From then on, the concurrent observation of a patient's health state to intelligent health appliances linked to mobile applications and the health service means that it is possible to obtain necessary health-related data, and the same can be used by a doctor to examine patients' health status and thereby arrange suitable treatment [11]. Radio-frequency identification (RFID) is wearable technology that can be allocated to a patient. Electronic health records (EHR) supply information gathered and placed in a database and then relocated to a doctor by a system administrator on their systems. They can utilise this information for various purposes, from examining collected information to developing innovative treatments [12].

1.3 NEED FOR IOT IN THE HEALTHCARE INDUSTRY

Before introducing IoT, patients' contacts with hospitals and doctors were inadequate, done with phone calls and text message communications. Therefore, there were no ways for hospitals and doctors to observe patients' health constantly and make suggestions as a result [13]. After the introduction of IoT-facilitated devices, there has been a drastic change in the healthcare industry. This technology has made possible the monitoring of patients remotely, creating opportunities to keep patients secure and well, and allowing physicians to deliver unbeatable care. Apart from these, the following are the reasons that demand the use of IoT in the healthcare industry [14].

1.3.1 FEWER PATIENT APPOINTMENTS AND MEDICATION ADHERENCE

Frequently, patients merely disregard the necessities of experts through folk medicines or medicine that associates suggest. But the solutions given by IoT are very accurate, and also tracks whether patients have adhered to medication as per the doctor's prescription. Moreover, the doctor can always observe and control the treatment progression of a patient [15].

1.3.2 SLOW TREATMENT PROCESS AND DELAYS IN HOSPITAL DISCHARGES

Even on ordinary days, hospitals do not have enough health workers for taking care of patients who have approached hospitals. The current pandemic has revealed this issue, increased this difficulty in recent times and demonstrated the disadvantages in the current healthcare sector. Added to this is a the need for competent medical and healthcare experts, more well-equipped rooms, etc. Incorporating IoT into the healthcare industry will improve and shorten the process of providing support significantly [16]. Further, IoT enabled technology can assist in taking care of the patients, improve the workflow, forecast patient influx during a pandemic time, etc.

1.3.3 UNDERFUNDING AND MISPLACEMENT OF RESOURCES

The modern healthcare industry is resource-intensive, and it will not be feasible to assemble such necessities forever [17]. This kind of situation exists more in African as well as Asian countries. IoT would considerably increase the sustainability of premises, hospitals, workforce, transportation, and the like [18].

1.4 USES OF IOT IN HEALTHCARE

IoT-enabled medical appliances monitor in the healthcare industry remotely as possible, discharges its services to maintain patients' safety and health and allows doctors to provide excellent care for patients. It also increases patients' commitment and happiness through frequent and convenient interactions with healthcare practitioners [19]. Besides, IoT helps monitor patients' health and aids in diminishing the length of stay in hospital and avoids unnecessary readmissions. IoT plays a significant role in reducing healthcare expenses considerably and promoting the outcomes of the treatment. IoT is unquestionably changing the healthcare industry by redesigning the area of IoT-enabled technologies and patient relations by providing health-related suggestions [20]. The application of IoT in the healthcare industry benefits different stakeholders, such as patients, people, healthcare professionals, hospitals, and insurance companies. The following are the benefits provided by IoT for various stakeholders.

1.4.1 Patients

IoT-enabled wearables such as smart watches, smart bands and other devices observe health-related aspects such as blood pressure, heartbeat rate, walking steps, sugar levels, etc., to provide individualised attention. These technologies can also be adjusted to repeat calorie burnt count, check appointments, variations in blood pressure, and much more [21]. IoT has modified peoples' lives in many aspects, particularly in aged patients, by allowing continuous checking of health situations. IoT has a great impact on the people who are living alone. They also observe any difficulties or deviations in the regular behaviour of an individual; the attentive instruments mail a signal to family members and healthcare service providers [22].

1.4.2 Physicians

IoT-powered wearable and other home-monitoring instruments help physicians to maintain the health of patients effectively. These instruments look after the patients' commitments to treatment arrangements or any other requirement for instant medicinal consideration. IoT facilitates medical practitioners to be more attentive and apply themselves to the patients dedicatedly [22]. Further, data collected from IoT-enabled instruments will assist medical practitioners to provide the finest medical treatment for patients and reach the projected results.

1.4.3 Hospitals

IoT-enabled instruments, devices are attached with sensors, are playing major roles in hospitals. Instruments capture the concurrent locations of healthcare utensils like defibrillators, smart beds, oxygen ventilators and pumps, wheelchairs, and other observing instruments. Moreover, the use of this technology also enables us to watch the medical staff at different locations. The risk from disease is the main concern for patients in hospitals. IoT-powered sanitation examining instruments assist in preventing patients from receiving infections [23]. IoT-enabled healthcare equipment also assists in managing the assets in the hospitals, like monitoring and controlling pharmacy inventory, and monitoring premises, like inspecting the temperature of the refrigerator, and maintaining and controlling the humidity and temperature in rooms.

1.4.4 HEALTH INSURANCE COMPANIES

IoT offers several opportunities for health insurance companies by connecting IoT-enabled intelligent equipment. Insurance companies can increase the amount of data collected through various health-monitoring devices. Thereby, it assists insurance companies during underwriting and claims settlement. The data collected from these instruments will enable insurance companies to identify fraudulent claims and discover possibilities for underwriting. Moreover, IoT-enabled equipment facilitates clarity between insurance companies and clients while assessing risk, underwriting, pricing, and settling claims [24]. Due to IoT-enabled technologies, patients can make accurate decisions in connection with different operation processes. Clients would have sufficient clarity of the original thought behind every result established and progression outcomes. Insurance companies may provide impetus to their clients for utilising and disseminating health-related data collected by IoT-enabled devices. They may also compensate clients for utilising IoT-enabled devices to keep checking their regular actions and follow up medication plans, thereby taking preventive health-related actions if needed. This would facilitate insurance companies to reduce claims considerably [25]. Utilising the data collected by these technologies, IoT-enabled technologies can also allow insurance companies to authenticate claims.

1.5 HOW IOT WORKS IN THE HEALTHCARE INDUSTRY

The development of health-related IoT technologies offers unimaginable services by processing millions of pieces of data. This large volume of data collected by IoT-enabled devices allows the possibility of transforming the healthcare industry with accurate outcomes [12]. IoT has built on a four-stage framework, and all four stages have been connected to collect the data in one stage, and the collected data will be processed in the second stage, thus providing the outcome at subsequent stages. Thus, the interconnected devices in the health care process send data to the hospitals; thereby it leads to better healthcare prospects.

IoT-enabled interconnected devices collect the necessary data in the first stage by using monitors, sensors, cameras, actuators, and other related devices. Normally, the sensors will send the data in analogue format. This analogue data must be collected and transformed to a digital format to facilitate further processing. After the data is transformed to digital format, it will be in pre-processed format; after that, it will be processed and standardised and sent to data storage or the cloud. Finally, the stored data will be analysed with advanced analytics methods to take effective and actionable business decisions. Thus, IoT has transformed the healthcare industry and ensured enhanced care for patients, better treatment outcomes, reduced treatment costs considerably and pipelined better process and workflows. Moreover, it improves the performance of healthcare service providers and increases the satisfaction of patients.

1.5.1 Benefits of IoT in the Healthcare Industry

IoT is changing the health sector drastically, and it is influencing society to move along with its applications and instruments. Thereby it facilitates people to interact with healthcare professionals for obtaining health-related solutions. Thus, IoT has given a new viewpoint as novel technologies have accommodated a combined healthcare system; consequently, the care offered is of a superior standard [26]. IoT in the healthcare industry operates with automation technologies with fewer errors. In recent times several hospitals have started to use IoT-enabled technologies to manage temperature, airflow, and humidity in operation theatres. Thus, the benefits IoT offer the health sector are countless. A few of the benefits generated by the IoT are as follows:

1.5.2 IoT Enhances the Capabilities of Preventive Medicine

With the help of data collected by IoT, doctors can comprehend patient's physical condition better and react as a result. The collected data permits doctors to observe patients' physical condition and warning signs and address problems with no delay. For these kinds of matters, neural network-enabled data analytics works better along with the vast usage of IoT [27].

1.5.3 Increased Mobility and Alertness of Hospital Staff

During the time of the pandemic, more patients required immediate healthcare support. At the same time, healthcare professionals were working beyond the limits of their ability. So, healthcare professionals require advanced technologies to monitor hundreds of patients concurrently [28]. With IoT-enabled tracking systems, healthcare professionals can make alterations instantly when serious changes occur in patients' health and rapidly find patients who need help and immediate assistance.

1.5.4 Accelerated Processing of Patient Data

Usually, doctors or healthcare professionals spend hours together processing various types of data manually, but for the same IoT will take a few minutes. In addition, IoT, incorporated with AI and ML, can offer possible medication alternatives [29].

1.5.5   Improved Drug Management and Better Adherence to Medicines

IoT plays a major role in the drug management and medicine adherence process. IoT-enabled applications help the doctors, medical professionals, healthcare service providers monitor the patients remotely and thereby helps monitor whether the patient has used the medicines; if not, healthcare service providers will call and advise the patients about the downsides of the same. Sometimes this type of process will be systemised [30].

1.5.6   Reduced Risk of Error and Inaccuracy due to the Human Factor

While doing sample tests, lab technicians or doctor may come up with incorrect results, leading to the wrong conclusion. Employing human factors in the healthcare service can lead to various serious problems. But these kinds of shortcomings can be avoided with the help of IoT [31]. IoT-enabled technologies will provide the utmost accuracy in diagnosing patients.

1.5.7   Secure Data Transfer to Doctors

As far as data transformation is concerned, it should be confidential, and no one should be able to see it with the exception of the attending physician. IoT enables the confidential transformation of data directly from one instrument to another [32].

1.6   SHORTCOMINGS OF IOT IN THE HEALTHCARE INDUSTRY

Even though IoT can be of huge advantage or benefit to the healthcare industry, some shortcomings must be tackled before implementing this fully. The shortcomings or challenges of using IoT-enabled instruments in the healthcare industry are as follows:

1.6.1   Safety and Security

Both safety and security remain major problems and discourage users from utilising IoT-enabled devices for healthcare and medical-related activities, as health-related data-monitoring devices can be hacked or breached. Disclosure of patients' confidential data about their physical condition and locality and interfering with sensor data can produce serious problems, which would counter the advantages of IoT [33].

1.6.2   Risk of System Failure

The breakdown or failure of systems hardware or power failure leading to the stoppage of sensors and other interconnected devices places the healthcare operations at risk. Further, omitting a regular software update may also be more dangerous than omitting a medical check-up [34].

1.6.3 INTEGRATION

There is no legal consensus or agreement about the usage of IoT protocol and standards, so equipment manufactured by various producers may not be the same and work well together. The lack of consistency and standardisation in quality prevents full incorporation of IoT in healthcare operations; as a result, it is limiting the potential effectiveness [35].

1.6.4 COST

Although IoT ensures minimise healthcare costs over an extended period of time, the cost incurred for its execution in hospitals and other medical institutions is very high. The cost incurred for staff training is also fairly high as it requires specialised trainers.

1.7 FUTURE OF HEALTHCARE WITH IOT TECHNOLOGY

The main reason for the increased usage of IoT-enabled technologies in the healthcare industry during the quarantine times is the shortage of doctors and healthcare service providers. The lack of human resources was managed intelligently by increasing the application of drones, aerial vehicles, smartphone applications for telemedicine, and remote technologies for follow-up with patients through various wearable devices, etc. The testing of unmanned aerial vehicles for related usage in the healthcare supply chain is already in the pipeline. Primarily, drones are utilised to transfer donor blood quickly from one place to another. In future, drones will be used to supply medicines to patients undergoing residence treatment. RFID is one of the latest IoT-enabled technologies that have supported a lot of the health sector, and it provides many benefits to the healthcare industry [36]. Thus, RFID helps to improve the functioning of IoT in healthcare solutions, and it will allow the incorporation of RFID-enabled technologies. By 2025, RFID-enabled technologies will be used in different fields, such as patient care, monitoring the hospital environment, and managing the inventory in medical institutions. Indeed, with high-speed broadband, well-equipped data analytics technology, along with technological developments, more participants have entered this market space; thus, the prospects for IoT have increased to create a constructive impact on the health sector [37].

Although IoT-enabled technologies in the healthcare industry were slower in the initial phase than other industries, its scope has now changed with the emergence of a new field called the Internet of Medical Things (IoMT). It is about to transform the healthcare industry along with smart and reliable technologies. Thus, it is ensuring the health and safety of the people in a cost-efficient way. All these data have proved the prospective outlook of IoT in the healthcare industry [38]. By supporting this, in recent years, the IoT market size has constantly been increasing due to the interests of new producers. Field experts have forecast that the market segment of wearable technology will reach about USD 74.03 billion by 2025; it was USD 27.91 billion in 2019. Wearable technology is considered as one of the essential technologies contributing to the healthcare industry, because it will launch new technologies to the market. Thus, patients can monitor their health by themselves [39]. Frost and Sullivan's analysis reported that the worldwide IoT market size would be USD 72.02 billion by 2021, at a CACR of 26.2%, and it was USD 22.5 billion in 2016. Contributing immense support to the healthcare industry, the IoT market is overflowing with various smart devices like smartphones, digital gadgets, wearables, medical and other monitors for observing the health condition in homes, society, hospital, or hospital surroundings connecting with the concurrent location, and providing telehealth, along with other services [40].

Additionally, the on-body segment is classified into two divisions: patients' health wearables and medicinal or clinical-grade wearables. Patients' health wearables – digital bands, wristbands, sports watches, and smart garments – contain consumer-grade devices for the wellness or health of the individual by tracking activities. Businesses operating in this segment include Samsung Medical, Fitbit, Redmi health, Misfit, and Withings. Clinical-grade wearables comprise synchronised devices and maintain platforms that are usually approved and certified by health regulatory bodies or authorities, such as the Indian Medical Association. Thus, it is clear that IoT and its role in the healthcare industry are enormous [37].

1.8 CONCLUSIONS

IoT is restoring the healthcare industry in a revolutionary way, as the populace has started to utilise IoT-enabled technologies for managing their health necessities. For instance, persons can use IoT-powered technologies to ring a bell about doctors' schedules, differences in blood pressure level, sugar level, calories burnt, distance walked, etc. One of the most significant segments of IoT in the health sector is monitoring patients' health by remote technology, where patients can be observed and prescribed from somewhere else. Concurrent location services are yet another benefit given by IoT, thus initiating a significant move towards the next stage of the health industry [41]. Using these real-time location services, medical practitioners can easily follow device locations, which decreases the time spent on this process. IoT-enabled smartphone usage is rising rapidly, and people have commenced using smartphone applications for doing anything. In the healthcare industry, smartphone applications will serve better to get better communications between patients and medical practitioners and their highly protected environment. An essential duty is for digital or smart health advisors and clinicians to work together while the healthcare industry is transforming towards an IoT-enabled environment. For the successful running of the IoT-enabled healthcare industry, suitable training and continuous feedback are essential for better and smart operation [42]. The conventional method of collecting patients' particulars, such as a pen and pad along with paper lying on the patients' bed, will not work anymore, because such information can be used only by limited people and may be lost or scrambled. IoT-enabled technology will work perfectly at this juncture as they provide stress-free data collection and management platforms on the devices. Thus, health-related data will be obtainable electronically, at any time, once safety and security provisions are met.

REFERENCES

1. Healthtech. "How is IoT Solving Pain Points in Healthcare?" Accessed October 12, 2020. www.healthtechzone.com/topics/healthcare/articles/2020/05/27/445511-how-iot-solving-pain-points-healthcare.htm.
2. Robinson. D. "Five Ways IoT Will Bring Healthcare into the 21st Century – Including Asthma Monitoring and Virtual Doctors." Accessed October 10, 2020. www.ns-healthcare.com/analysis/iot-in-healthcare/.
3. Masilamani. "How IoT Applications Have Transformed the Way Healthcare Sector Works." Accessed October 11, 2020. https://blog.contus.com/iot-healthcare-applicati ons-benefits/.
4. Orekhova, K. "The Role of IoT in Healthcare Industry: Benefits and Use Cases." Accessed October 13, 2020. www.cleveroad.com/blog/iot-in-healthcare.
5. Prashant, A. "7 Amazing Use Cases of IoT in Healthcare." Accessed October 13, 2020. www.pratititech.com/blog/7-amazing-use-cases-of-iot-in-healthcare.
6. Businesswire. "Global IoT in Healthcare Market by Component, by Connectivity, by Application, by Geography and the Impact of COVID-19 (2020–2025)." Accessed October 15, 2020. www.businesswire.com/news/home/20200828005105/en/Global-IoT-in-Healthcare-Market-2020-2025-Demand-Growing-Exponentially-at-a-CAGR-of-18---ResearchAndMarkets.com.
7. Mordor Intelligence. "Internet of Things (IoT) In Healthcare Market – Growth, Trends, and Forecast (2020–2025)." Accessed October 15, 2020. www.mordorintelligence. com/industry-reports/internet-of-things-in-healthcare-market.
8. The Daily Chronicle. "Internet of Things (IoT) in Healthcare Market Growth Insights 2020-by Key Players, Research by Top Trends, Revenue, Share, Business Size Forecast to 2024." Accessed October 11, 2020. https://thedailychronicle.in/news/2270736/inter net-of-things-iot-in-healthcare-market-growth-insights-2020-by-key-players-research-by-top-trends-revenue-share-business-size-forecast-to-2024/.
9. Ray, P.P. "Understanding the role of internet of things towards smart e-healthcare ser-vices." *Biomedical Research*, 28(4), 2016, 38–52.
10. eSparkBiz. "The Role of IoT in the Healthcare Industry." Accessed October 29, 2020. https://theiotmagazine.com/the-role-of-iot-in-the-healthcare-industry-ba361678da7a.
11. Biz4intellia. "Benefits of IoT Applications and Gadgets for the Healthcare Industry." Accessed October 29, 2020. www.biz4intellia.com/blog/applications-of-iot-in-healthcare/.
12. Wipro. "What Can IoT Do for Healthcare?." Accessed October 29, 2020. www.wipro. com/en-IN/business-process/what-can-iot-do-for-healthcare-/#:~:text=IoT enables healthcare professionals to,and reach the expecte.
13. Puresoftware. "The Need of Internet of Things (IoT) in Healthcare." Accessed October 21, 2020. https://puresoftware.com/the-need-of-internet-of-things-iot-inhealthcare
14. Markets and Markets. "IoT in Healthcare Market." Accessed October 29, 2020. www.marketsandmarkets.com/Market-Reports/iot-healthcare-market-160082804. html#:~:text=%5B307%20Pages%20Report%5D%20The%20global,21.0%25%20 during%20the%20forecast%20period.
15. Medical Device Network. "Bringing the Internet of Things to Healthcare." Accessed October 29, 2020. www.medicaldevice-network.com/comment/bringing-internet-things-healthcare/.
16. Finoit. "The Role of IoT in Healthcare: Applications and Implementation." Accessed November 9, 2020. www.finoit.com/blog/the-role-of-iot-in-healthcare-space/.

17. Digiteum. "Benefits of Using IoT in the Healthcare Industry." Accessed November 4, 2020. www.digiteum.com/iot-benefits-healthcare-industry#.

18. Inieke, O. "Internet of Things in Healthcare: The Social, Ethical, Legal & Professional Implications." (Preprints). www.preprints.org/manuscript/202001.0359/v1.

19. Abhinav, S. "6 Reasons Why Healthcare Needs the Internet of Things (IoT)." Accessed November 9, 2020. https://hitconsultant.net/2017/11/03/internet-things-digital-future-value-based-care/#.X7DK5XQzbIU.

20. Sheldon, A. "IoT in Healthcare: Benefits, Challenges and Applications." Accessed November 8, 2020. www.valuecoders.com/blog/technology-and-apps/iot-in-healthcare-benefits-challenges-and-applications/.

21. Intellectsoft. "IoT in Healthcare: Benefits, Use Cases, Challenges, and Future." accessed November 10, 2020. www.intellectsoft.net/blog/iot-in-healthcare/.

22. Nasrullah, P. "Internet of Things Healthcare Applications Benefits and Challenges" Accessed November 12, 2020. www.peerbits.com/blog/internet-of-things-healthcare-applications-benefits-and-challenges.html.

23. Techutzpah. "Internet of Things (IoT) Healthcare Benefits." Accessed November 10, 2020. https://theiotmagazine.com/internet-of-things-iot-healthcare-benefits-2aae663c5c79.

24. Cprime. "Benefits of Internet of Things for hospitals and healthcare." Accessed November 11, 2020. https://archer-soft.com/blog/benefits-internet-things-hospitals-and-healthcare.

25. Skelia. "5 Benefits Of Using IoT In Healthcare That Outweigh The Challenges It Presents." accessed November 11, 2020. https://skelia.com/articles/5-benefits-of-using-iot-in-healthcare-that-outweigh-the-challenges-it-presents/.

26. Osetskyi, V. "IoT in Healthcare: Use Cases, Trends, Advantages, and Disadvantages." Accessed November 9, 2020. https://dzone.com/articles/iot-in-healthcare-use-cases-trends-advantages-and.

27. Elizabeth, M. "4 Big Benefits of the "Internet of Things" In Healthcare." Accessed November 10, 2020. www.jmark.com/4-big-benefits-of-the-internet-of-things-in-healthcare/.

28. Validic. "Guest Blog: The Benefits of IoT in Healthcare." Accessed November 10, 2020. https://validic.com/guest-blog-the-benefits-of-iot-in-healthcare/.

29. Ardas. "Top 7 Benefits of IoT for Healthcare and Wellness." Accessed November 10, 2020. https://ardas-it.com/7-benefits-of-iot-for-people-in-the-healthcare-wellness-industry-ardas-it.

30. Kot, J. "4 benefits of Internet of Things for healthcare." Accessed November 10, 2020. https://concisesoftware.com/4-benefits-of-internet-of-things-for-healthcare/.

31. xcube Labs. "5 Key Benefits of IoT for HealthCare Organizations." Accessed November 10, 2020. www.xcubelabs.com/blog/benefits-iot-in-healthcare/.

32. Raut, P. "Internet of Things in Healthcare Industry: Benefits and Challenges." Accessed November 11, 2020. https://yourstory.com/mystory/internet-of-things-in-healthcare-industry-benefits.

33. Maxim, C. "3 Challenges of Healthcare Internet of Things (IoT) Performance Testing." Accessed November 10, 2020. www.google.com/search?q=hitconsultant.net%2F2019%2F05%2F21%2F3-challenges-of-healthcare-internet-of-things-iot-performance.

34. Invma. "Patient-centred: The Challenges and Promises of IoT for Healthcare." Accessed November 11, 2020. https://invma.co.uk/knowledge-hub/blog/challenges-and-promises-of-IoT-for-healthcare.

35. Cdnsol. "IoT in Healthcare: Benefits, Challenges, and Applications." accessed November 11, 2020. https://www.cdnsol.com/blog/iot-in-healthcare-benefits-challenges-and-applications/.
36. Zeadally, S., Siddiqui, F., Baig, Z. and Ibrahim, A. "Smart healthcare: Challenges and potential solutions using internet of things (IoT) and big data analytics," *PSU Research Review*, 4(2), 2016, 149–168. https://doi.org/10.1108/PRR-08-2019-0027.
37. Singh, C. "What is the Future Scope of IoT in Healthcare?" Accessed November 12, 2020. www.appventurez.com/blog/iot-healthcare-future-scope/.
38. Omnia-Health. "IoT is the Future of Healthcare." Accessed November 12, 2020. https://insights.omnia-health.com/technology/iot-future-healthcare.
39. Chouffani, R. "Future of IoT in Healthcare Brought into Sharp Focus." Accessed November 12, 2020. https://internetofthingsagenda.techtarget.com/feature/Can-we-expect-the-Internet-of-Things-in-healthcare.
40. Mordor Intelligence. "Internet of Things (Iot) In Healthcare Market – Growth, Trends, And Forecast (2020–2025)." Accessed November 12, 2020. www.mordorintelligence.com/industry-reports/internet-of-things-in-healthcare-market.
41. Tech Wire Asia. "How IoT Solutions Are Defining the Future of the Healthcare Industry." Accessed November 13, 2020. https://techwireasia.com/2019/11/how-iot-solutions-are-defining-the-future-of-the-healthcare-industry/.
42. Webdesk. "IoT in Healthcare Expectations for 2020." Accessed November 13, 2020. www.digitalinformationworld.com/2020/02/iot-in-healthcare-expectations-for-2020.html.

2 IoT Devices for Measuring Pulse Rates and ECG Signals

Bhagyashri Pandurangi R.
Department of Electronics and Communication Engineering
KLS Gogte Institute of Technology

Ashwini R. Hirekodi
Osteos India Pvt. Ltd.
Mahantesh Nagar, Belagavi

CONTENTS

DOI: 10.1201/9781003146087-3

Technologies have been improving day by day, where all the work is being done digitally. Health specialists and doctors still use old methods of storing the data, with manually recording, leading to many errors. This can be improved with a process where we can store the readings of vital parameters such as pulse and electrocardiogram (ECG) digitally. This step avoids errors encountered due to the manual entry of the data in the electronic medical record (EMR) system and related applications. The pulse readings will be published to the Node.JS application once the patient ID is received. The Node. JS then stores the readings to the MongoDB database along with the patient's ID. The key objective of this automatic update of pulse or ECG measurements of patients is to prevent any errors caused due to the manual entry of the pulse or ECG readings. The data of any patient can be readily accessed anytime through the EMR system.

2.1 INTRODUCTION

Vital parameters like pulse and ECG readings of a patient are measured using sensors connected to a single board computer such as Raspberry Pi. The Raspberry Pi has been chosen for collecting sensor data as it has all the necessary resources and a powerful CPU to run multiple applications on a standalone board. The Internet of Things (IoT) has always been more essential in health, where using the right technique to regularly check up on health is no longer an issue. Using IoT, there is no need for routine visits to doctors. With the help of IoT, doctors can keep track of our health records and monitor us from any part of the world and suggest what has to be done for recovery. With all this improvement, we can have IoT robotic arms, which can perform operations on us under the guidance of doctors. In this chapter, we show how the pulse and ECG of a person can be stored and later accessed from the database at any given time and any given place.

Kevin Ashton was the first person to initiate IoT in 1999 [1]. This is the physical transmission web where billions of data are collected from various devices and transformed into usable information [2]. With unparalleled growth, by 2020 we could connect to 50 billion devices through IoT telecommunication [3]. IoT can be used in the medical field to monitor patients from any place at any time. This system can be used for patients who need continuous monitoring of their health.

An organized review of various mobile medical management has been seen from their point of view [4]. ECG observation service through cloud-based services was introduced [5].

A bridge was established between the "digital" and the "real" world by IoT. The gadgets are coupled to the cloud and generate individual recognition over the internet [6]. Vital parameters like pulse and ECG readings of the patient are checked using the sensors connected to the Raspberry Pi. Raspberry Pi has been used as it can interact with the outside world and transfer data. The transferred data is stored in a private cloud. Here the obtained data is in the form of analog output. The ADS1115 is a 16-bit ADC chip used to convert data from analog to digital, obtained from the sensors. The digital data obtained are sent to the Raspberry Pi where the Python application runs, and the samples are sent to the Node.JS webserver, an open-source cloud. With the growth in production technologies, gadgets have become tiny, with less electricity consumption and reduced costs [7].

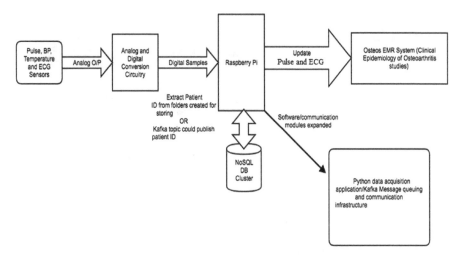

FIGURE 2.1   High-level architecture for vital signs integration.

Figure 2.1 shows how the pulse is converted and sent to the cloud. MySQL is used for storing the data that is received from sampling. The digital samples that are received are updated every time a patient comes for a follow-up. These digital samples are then set aside in the MongoDB database beside the patient ID. The facts obtained from patients are stored under their respective IDs. After submitting the form, pulse and ECG values will be sent to the controller via REST API and stored in the respective patient's collection in the MongoDB database. When the doctors need any health details of the patients, they just need to enter the patient's ID, and the EMR trigger start pulse and ECG measurements that are updated in the WebSocket can be obtained. WebSocket stores all necessary data in a server where it can be easily accessed.

The devices used for connections are as shown in Figure 2.2. (a) ADS1115 is a 16-bit analog to digital converter used to send digital samples to the database. (b) A pulse sensor is used for checking the pulse, which has three wires. The red wire is connected to VCC, the black is connected to the ground and the purple is connected to channel number 0 of ADS1115. (c) Echo cardiogram is used so that a graphical representation of the heartbeat can be obtained.

2.1.1   SENSOR FOR PULSE

The sensor that is used for the checking pulse is very simple. There are two sides; one side of it is LED, the other side is circuitry. The circuitry is used for the noise cancellation and amplification of pulses. The LED is used to check the pulse placed on the vein of a fingertip or an ear tip. A heart rate monitor (HRM) is used for measuring or displaying the pulse, which can be checked at the time or can be used for later use. HRM uses the technique of recording the pulse rate while the patient is performing various types of exercises. HRM is used for measuring ECG, where the

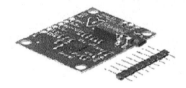

a). ADS1115

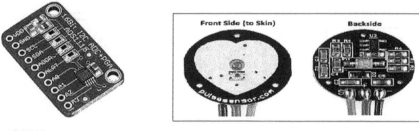

b). Pulse Sensor

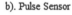

c). Echo cardiogram chip

FIGURE 2.2   Devices used (a) ADS1115 ADC, (b) Pulse Sensor, (c) Echocardiogram chip.

electrical heart monitor is referred to. The electrical monitor consists of a transmitter and receiver. The transmitter is used to monitor ECG whenever a heartbeat is detected, and the receiver is used to display the current heartbeat. A chest strap is attached to the patient from which readings will be transmitted – a simple or unique coded signal. The medium used for transmitting these can be Connect time, ANT, or different ineffective transmission connections. Eavesdropping and crosstalk interference can be prevented if we try using a newer technology so that one signal cannot be used by the other. Polar 5.1 kHz transmission telecommunication is usable under water, whereas both Connect time and Ant+ have a 2.4GHz transmission band that is not suitable.

The LED's light should directly fall on the vein. Blood will be flowing in the veins only if there is inflate in the heart. So, when observation is done on blood flow, heartbeat can be checked too. To determine heartbeat, the ambient light sensor detects the flow of blood, making the reflecting light lighter; this change in the received light is analyzed and determines heart rate over time. In this chapter, the sensor that checks pulse acts as a pulse antenna for Raspberry Pi. Even though chest straps are efficient, wrist-based heart rate monitors, which have been introduced recently, show high-efficiency rates up to 95%, although they may show an error of 30% if operated for a few minutes. Devices with digital readings show decreasingly accurate results over a period, especially underwater. Digital readings have lower heart rate variability currently. Apple launched the HRV facts assembly in 2018 to observe their gadgets.

2.1.2 ELECTROCARDIOGRAM CHIP

The method of collecting electric signals produced by the heart is called electrocardiography or ECG. The psychological state can be better understood with this, along with the level of physiological arousal one is experiencing. The cause of an increase in physiological arousal is often misattributed. Many things are unknown about the happenings in the human body. The important elements of an ECG are the QRS complex, which measures the change of the ventricles, the T wave, which measures the repolarization of the ventricles, and the P wave, which measures the depolarization of the atria.

In every heartbeat, a systematic sequence of depolarization starts from the sinoatrial node with the pacesetter cell, disperses all around the atrium, and sends the atrioventricular node into the bunch of Purkinje threads, dispersing below and to the left all around the ventricles. The singular ECG tracing is obtained due to the systematic design of depolarization. An ECG gives experts a horde of details about the infrastructure of the heart and the consequences of the electric conduction system. The size and position of the heart chambers and the heart rhythm can be measured by ECG. Also, any damage in the heart muscles or conduction structure, the effect of medicine on the heart, and the response of implants in the heart can be observed.

A coordinate of electrodes is associated with an important unit that records ECGs by the machines. Before digital readings, equivalent computer data is acquired where the gesture masses a motor to imprint the broadcast onto paper. Now, analog-to-digital transformers are used to transform the pulse of the heart into a digital gesture in ECGs. ECG instruments are now transferable and often incorporate a monitor, console, and composer. Recently we have seen a lot of improvement in electrocardiography, where smaller devices are used to track health in the form of smartwatches and fitness trackers. These compact devices frequently depend on only two electrodes to carry a single lead. There is accessibility of compact six-gadgets.

The procedure for ECG documentation is guarded and pain-free. The instruments are electrified with safety features that include bonded (ground) lead.

Other characteristics are:

- Defibrillation safety: ECG used in medical care is always connected to the person who needs to be brought around, making the heartbeat normal. ECG needs to keep itself safe from this origin of power.
- Conductor performance is the same as defibrillation performance, where voltage safety is up until 18,000 volts.
- Typically, 50–60 Hz mains power is used to reduce common-mode interference called the right leg driver, an additional circuitry.
- ECG voltages for the whole body are very small. Low noise circuits and instrumentation amplifiers are low voltage necessitates.
- Simultaneous lead recordings: Current models can record multiple leads compared to the old models, whereas old models could record each lead sequentially.

Nowadays, ECG instruments have self-explanation algorithms. This investigation considered characteristics such as the PR interval, QT interval, corrected QT (QTc) interval, PR axis, QRS axis, rhythm and many more. The output obtained from these self-explanation algorithms is regarded as preparation until it is approved by expert interpretation. Despite the advances in the computer field, misinterpretation of readings is still a big problem that can lead to clinical mismanagement.

2.1.3   RATE AND RHYTHM OF ECG

Heart rate, like other vital signs such as respiratory and blood pressure, changes with age. Normally, the heart rate is the rate at which the senatorial node where the electrical shock is given for a patient to get a normal heart rate is depolarized as it depolarizes the heart. The normal heart rate of adults is from 60 and 100bpm (normocardic), but in children it is excessive. A pulse rate that is less than the normal is known as "bradycardic" (<60 in elders), while higher than normal is known as "tachycardia" (>100 in elders). These complications happen in a person when there is simultaneous action between atria and ventricles, the heart rate must be mentioned as atrial and ventricular (e.g., the ventricular estimate in ventricular fibrillation is 300–600bpm, whereas the estimate of atrial is stable when it is between 60 to 100 and faster if it is 100 to 150). Normal sinus rhythm (NSR) is the normal physiological term for the resting heart. NSR generates the average sample of P wave, QRS complex, and T wave. In general, cardiac arrhythmia is a deviation from NSR. Thus, we have to know whether there is sinus rhythm in ECG interpretation. When P waves and QRS complexes appear as 1-to-1 which means the P waves cause the QRS complex is the main decision for sinus rhythm that is to be considered. Once we figure out whether the sinus rhythm is present or absent, the one further thing to be considered is rate. In this, the sinus rhythm occurs either due to P wave or QRS complexes following are 1-to-1. If the heart rate is rapidly increasing, it is known as sinus tachycardia, and if, by chance, the rate is rapidly decreasing, then it is sinus bradycardia. If the interpretation is not sinus rhythm, checking the rhythm is important before considering the next step.

Some arrhythmias with different characters:

- In atrial fibrillation, P waves are absent with "irregularly irregular" QRS complexes.
- In atrial flutter, the main thing is a "sawtooth" pattern with QRS complexes.
- In ventricular flutter, the hallmark is a sine wave pattern.
- In ventricular tachycardia, P waves are absent with wide QRS complexes and increased heart rate.

Determining rate and rhythm is very important when considering the next steps.

2.1.4   DIAGNOSIS

Based on ECG, we can make diagnoses and findings. Different pattern diagnoses can be undertaken. For example, in atrial fibrillation, an irregularly irregular QRS complex can be found in the absence of P waves; but, after examining, we can see that other findings too are present, like a bunch of separate pieces that change the shape of QRS complexes. This is the main reason why ECG is considered only for the heartbeat and not for other diagnoses. For example: In hyperkalemia, examination of peaked T waves is not good enough, but also diagnosis of blood potassium is to be measured and verified. Conversely, if there is the presence of peaked T waves, extended QRS complexes, and dropping of P waves, then the invention of hyperkalemia acts in accordance with ECG.

2.1.5　ADS1115 Analog to Digital Converter

In microcontrollers, when we want to convert analog to digital or want higher accuracy ADC, the ADS1115 has 16-bit precision at 860samples/second over I2C. The ADS1115 chip can be used as four transmission ends to end input medium or two dissimilar mediums. Increasing the smaller single/dissimilar gesture to full range even includes a program manager profit amplifier, up to x16. ADC is super easy to use, estimating a wide span of waves and runs from 2V–5V power/logic. It is an important universal resolution 16-bit converter. The other technical data of these chips are:

* Large reservoir: 2.0V–5.5V.
* Less charge intake: continuous mode: only 150µA single-shot mode: auto shut-down.
* Programmable fact estimate: 8 SPS to 860 SPS.
* Interior low-drift voltage reference.
* Interior oscillator.
* Interior PGA.
* I2C interface: pin-selectable addresses.
* Four single-ended or two different inputs.
* Programmable reference.
* This board/chip uses I2C 7-bit addresses between 0x48-0x4b, selectable with jumpers.

2.2　LITERATURE SURVEY

Researchers have worked on this subject for a long time. Here is a summary of the related work.

A project by Shola Usha Rani, Antony Ignations, BhavaVyasaHari, et al. [8] was proposed to gather the readings of various important indications of patients, and later to send the readings to the doctor or the individual about the health condition. In this project, MQTT communication is used to send the data to the cloud platform. The patient's vital sense is transmitted with the help of the pictorial representation.

In another project, Mehmet Tastan [9], a wearable sensor is used to keep track of the patient's heartbeat and blood level. The patient who is in a critical health situation can be continuously monitored using this technique. Suppose there is a fluctuation in the patient's health levels. In that case, the information/details of his health conditions are received by one of their household people or the consultant through email or Twitter notifications. This project aims to give medical treatment as soon as possible in case of heart diseases. Therefore, the survival chances of a patient are increased.

Syed Misbahuddin, Junaid Ahmed Zubairi, Abdul Rahman Alahdal, et al. [10] proposed the structure for the injured person of mass destruction who was almost treated. MEDTOC is a real-time ingredient used for integrated answers. The proposed system sends real-time details of the affected victims to the doctor or the central database about their health condition even before the patient's arrival. Medical staff can prepare for the necessary treatment and operate as soon as the patient arrives. The patient's data, which is transferred, is stored without the identification of the patient. But this project can only be useful if the disaster area has a cellular network. If cellular networks are having issues, then different Wi-Fi connections will be utilized in the coming time. In a project by Dvarte Dias, Joao Paulo Silva Cunha [11], wearable devices are all based on broadband networks, which are only helpful if the connection is good. As they mentioned in their paper, the system will not be helpful, in countries like France, where there is less internet usage.

This can be further improved by using dry electrodes, which may cause discomfort on the skin. To store all the data in the long run in a cloud-based database.

2.3   HARDWARE AND SOFTWARE PLATFORM

This section has a detailed review of the hardware and the software implementation of the project.

2.3.1   HARDWARE PLATFORM

Figure 2.3 shows the hardware implementation of pulse sensor, ADS1115 ADC, to convert analog to digital readings. Raspberry Pi 4 is used to connect pulse sensors and then send data to private clouds. The three wires of the sensors are for Signal(S), Vcc (3-5V), and GND. In this project, the sensor is powered by 3.3V, and the sign which is attached is associated with Raspberry Pi from the ADS1115 ADC module since Raspberry Pi, of course, cannot peruse analog voltage. The following are the associations accomplished for beat sensor:

- Signal pin of heartbeat sensor - > A0 of ADC Module
- Vcc pin of heartbeat sensor - > 3.3V of Raspberry
- GND pin of heartbeat sensor - > GND of Pi
- Tx of RPI-> Rx of RPI
- GND of ADC module - > GND of RPI
- VCC of ADC Module - > +5v of RPI
- SCL and SDA of ADC module - > SCL and SDA of RPI

Pulse sensor and ECG are connected to the Raspberry Pi through ADS1115. The analog readings from sensors such as pulse and ECG are converted to digital samples before being consumed by the collector application running on Raspberry Pi.

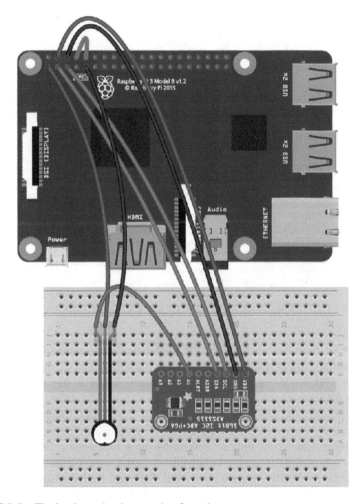

FIGURE 2.3 The hardware implementation for pulse sensor.

Pulse sensors and ECG are used for checking the heartbeat of the person. Figure 2.4 shows the connections done using ECG and pulse sensors. The connections shown in the figure are made using jumping wires, where ECG is connected to channel 2 as the pulse sensor is connected to channel 1. Here the ADC used is the 16-bit which is ultra-small and has low power. The consumption of power is less. Raspberry Pi is a minimal effort, Mastercard sized single-board PC dependent on ARM cortex design. Raspberry Pi is a decent decision for creating IoT undertakings and applications with a force processor, working velocity, and remote capacities.

2.3.2 RASPBERRY PI 4

The Raspberry Pi is a development from a single board PC created in the United Kingdom by the Raspberry Pi Foundation to advance knowledge of required software

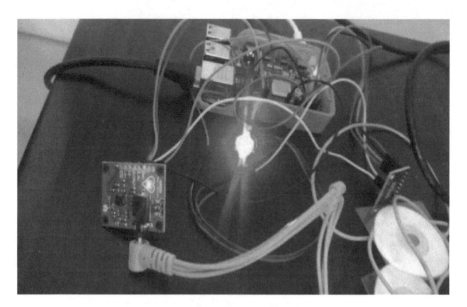

FIGURE 2.4   Real-time connections using ADS1115 with a pulse sensor and ECG.

engineering in the classrooms. The first model that was created became famous and was undoubtedly bestselling in the market for software systems. It is generally used for research work, e.g. tracking climatic changes, that is super easy and more convenient than any other project work. It does not include main components (for example, consoles and mice) or cases. Whatever the reason, the exaggeration has been in memory for a few formal and unofficial groups. Raspberry Pi, 4 Model B, was released in June 2019 with a 1.5 GHz 64-piece four center ARM Cortex-A72 processor, on-board 802.11ac Wi-Fi, Bluetooth 5, full gigabit Ethernet (throughput not restricted), two USB 2.0 ports, two USB 3.0 ports, and double screen support employing a couple of miniaturized scales (HDMI Type D) ports for up to 4K goal.

The connection between Raspberry Pi and ADC is checked using the pseudo command to know the interfacing between two devices. In Figure 2.5, 48 is the port number that is being used for displaying the result. The port representation is given as 08*40. Once you get the port started, interfacing is done, and the analog data that is carried is sent to a private cloud.

2.3.3   SOFTWARE PLATFORM

The software used in this project is Linux, which uses Python code to run sensors. To check the pulse, we write a code in which we specify all the required parameters. For getting the analog output of the pulse sensor, the ADC module is interfaced via I2C communication. The upper peak and lower peak of the pulse is to be found. Then the difference between the peak points is taken to convert it into BPM. The simple crude yield is sent, and BPM is sent to the sequential port, perused from preparing IDE for additional procedures. Here we have interconnected the ADC chip through I2C

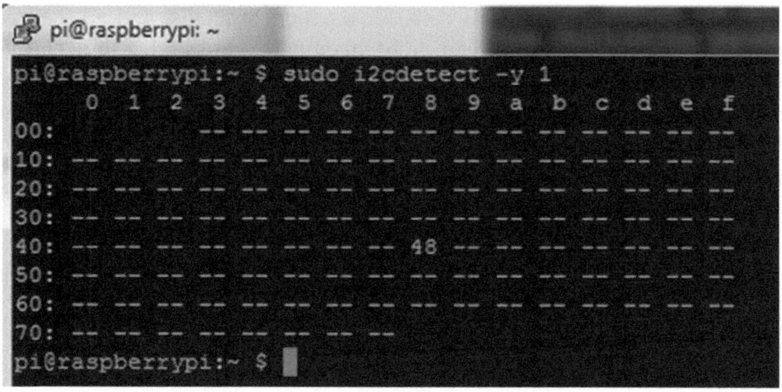

FIGURE 2.5   Detecting the interface between devices.

correspondence to get a simple yield of a heartbeat sensor. We locate the top pinnacle and bottom in the wake of getting crude simple yield from the beat sensor. And afterwards, discover the distinction of duration in two pinnacle focuses and afterwards converting rates in BPM. Furthermore, we send the crude, simple yield and BPM to sequential port, which is perused from handling IDE for additional procedures.

2.3.4   MySQL Database

MySQL is an open-source relational database management system. It serves as temporary storage of digital samples from sensors in real time before presenting their aggregated reading to the patient EMR front-end module. Eventually, the aggregated values will be stored in the cloud database (MongoDB) for patient medical history and continuous monitoring purposes. This database is used to store all the digital data received from the samples and are updated frequently whenever a patient comes for a visit. This data is stored under the patient ID so that to check the data becomes easy for medical staff. MySQL is developed and can be established through this code; however, it is usually established in a parallel bunch compared to uncommon customizations that are essential.

2.3.5   PhpMyAdmin

To communicate with MySQL, we write the code in PHP used to deal with the organization with the requirements of an internet browser. It uses different types of errands, for example, creating, changing, and deleting databases, tables, fields, or columns; finding the results for SQL explanation; or ignoring clients and consents. The product, accessible in 78 dialects, is maintained by the phpMyAdmin Project.

2.3.6   Webserver

The webserver used is Node.JS, a distributed SaaS-based cloud application interacting with front-end patient medical record systems. It is an open-source communicating server. Node.JS is used when staff calls for a patient's details, and all the updated readings are displayed on the screen. Subsequently, Node.JS talks to a "JavaScript all over" world view, bringing everything web application upgrading around a single coding language, differentiated to vary dialects for server- and customer-side contents.

The database program that is used for the cross-staging of records is MongoDB. Assigned to a NoSQL database program, MongoDB employs JSON-like records with optional developments. MongoDBInc introduces MongoDB.

2.3.7 ALGORITHMIC CODE OF PULSE SENSOR

Step 1: Import Adafruit_ADS1115, serial and time packages.

Step 2: Initialize all parameters where the pulse's peak and trough are set to 512.

Step 3: Interval between successive heartbeats is to be set as 600mS.

Step 4: Specify channel number 0 of ADS1115 for pulse sensor.

Step 5: Beats per minute is to be the ratio of 60000 by running total.

Step 6: The first beat of the pulse is true, and the second beat is to be given as false and vice versa alternatively.

Step 7: Time hopping is to be given as th = amp/2 + T.

Step 8: If there is no heartbeat, then "no beat found" is displayed.

Step 9: Sleeping time for beat is given as 0.05.

2.3.8 ALGORITHMIC CODE FOR ECG

Step 1: Import NumPy, pandas, neurokit, seaborn and ADS1115 packages.

Step 2: Initialize the parameters.

Step 3: Channel number 1 is to be specified for ECG.

Step 4: As it is a graphical representation, the epoch is set for 700mS, and the onset is -100.

Step 5: To get the data, the RR_max interval and baseline difference are to be considered.

Step 6: Data is then converted into a data frame.

2.3.9 ALGORITHMIC CODE FOR NODE.JS

Step 1: As this is a child process, we need to call the HTTPS server.

Step 2: Spawn is used in a webserver to call the Python code stored in Raspberry Pi.

Step 3: HTTPS webserver is then created for the request that is made.

Step 4: Content type is used to write Head response.

Step 5: Listen to the response that is sent.

2.4   RESULT AND PERFORMANCE ANALYSIS

The method is used so that patients can keep track of their health condition regularly. So that whenever there are any issues, they can contact their doctors as soon

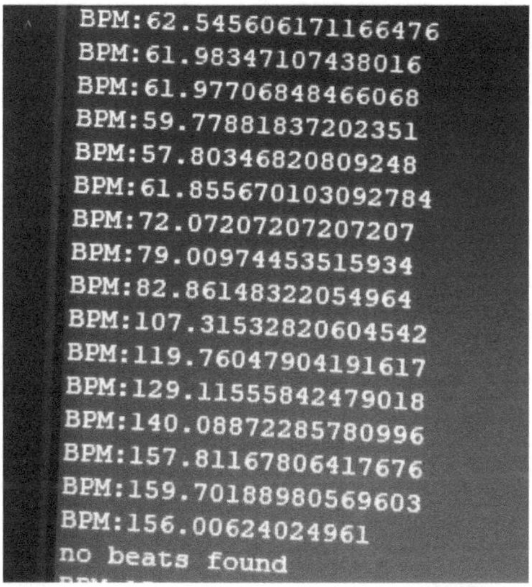

FIGURE 2.6   The readings of pulse on the cloud.

as possible. Even doctors can get reports from the MongoDB database by giving the patient's ID, which is stored when the patient comes for a check-up. When the patient ID is entered, the EMR triggers and readings are updated in the WebSocket. Compared to other devices, the proposed system can get readings to the doctor faster and is more accurate. Everything the patient originates to for check-up data remains acquired then is kept for almost a year.

Figure 2.6 shows the reading of a pulse sensor displayed on Raspberry Pi stored on a private cloud. Later the average of these readings is taken for displaying the pulse sensor. Whenever a beat is found, the pulse is measured and when there is no response from the person, then "no beat found" is displayed.

A database is an accumulation of data organized, usually stowed, then opened by a processor. Complicated records are frequently industrialized, employing approved projects then demonstrating methodologies. The database management system (DBMS) is a software program that interacts through end-users, requests, and itself to seize, observe, and analyze the data. The DBMS covers the central facilities given to managing the database. Database, the DBMS, then related requests are collectively referred to by the "database system". Often the period "database" remains second-hand to the DBMS, the database scheme, or a request related by the database slackly.

The patient's details are stored under the patient's ID. The database is in Excel form where name, age, weight and cellular number are mentioned. Medical information can only be accessed if the doctor or medical staff knows the password that is given. Only medical staff and doctors who are in charge of the patient can go through the medical history. The distributed notification message broker sends notifications between the applications running on Raspberry Pi and the EMR front-end web-based UI. The nurse who checks the patient's pulse will trigger the Node.

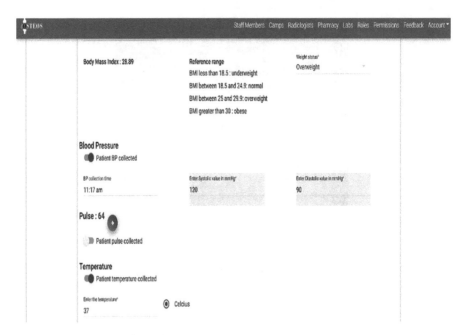

FIGURE 2.7   Node.JS webserver of EMR front-end.

JS server by clicking the arrow button, which is added in front of the pulse field. In response, Node.JS will send the calculated pulse reading received from the Python pulse sensor application to the EMR application and stored in the pulse field. With all other readings, the pulse value will be submitted and stored in the MongoDB database. As shown in Figure 2.7, the pulse is counted for 60 seconds. The best hardware for the EMR to setting up, customization and training.

The reading of ECG is displayed on the webserver from where the doctor gets all heartbeat information is being measured. The average efficiency of the ECG signal is 99%. An electrodermal activity sensor is used to check the human emotional level, and a photosensor is used to check changes that happen due to blood flow in the skin. The patient can also have access to this information if he knows the ID with which it is stored. Every time the patient comes to a check-up, information is acquired and stored as long as required. The storage capacity of the cloud is 1GB to 10GB. Discovery proceedings return a dict containing starts then periods of apiece individual occasion. Now, it accurately detects lone single occasions. Formerly, we were going to cut our information rendering toward that incident. The created period's purpose is a tilt having ages of data consistent with individual events. As we are taking only a single event, we will choose the 0th component of that lean.

Node.JS has an integral HTTP component, allowing Node.JS to transfer data over the hypertext transfer protocol (HTTP). The HTTP component cannot create an HTTP server that heeds to server ports and answers the client. Node.JS is an open-source, cross-platform, back-end, JavaScript runtime atmosphere that executes JavaScript code outside a web browser. Node.JS lets developers use JavaScript to write command-line tools and server-side scripting running scripts server-side to produce dynamic web page content before the page is sent to the user's web browser.

2.5 CONCLUSION AND FUTURE WORK

There are many ways of communication between patients and doctors and, by this method, they can not only communicate but can simultaneously track if the patient's health can be maintained. The stored data can be accessed easily by doctors and nurses just by entering the patient's ID. By using this method, the errors that occur while manually entering the data can be reduced. The readings can be accessed by medical staff and the patient only if the ID is known. The personal information of the patient is kept highly confidential using all the necessary steps. Patients having heart issues will be given great help with this device.

This can be further improved by adding more parameters like blood pressure, blood sugar, temperature and others. Even GPS can be used where data can be directly sent to a patient's ID and mailed to the doctor so continuous checking of the webserver can be reduced. The platform can easily be extended and/or integrated for conducting online consultations remotely using telehealth platforms. The patient's vital signs data collected on this platform could be used for ML and AI-based prediction models for early detection of specific diseases. Later all the required data is displayed on the mobile screen. Because the market is more aware of the possibilities, there has been an increase in investment of R&D, and improved products that can be obtained in shops; with any luck, this will intensify the growth of the market in the coming year.

The main three features required in the device knowledge zone are extended period constancy, resiliency, and biocompatibility. Being in electronics development, smaller sensors are also to be developed to increase the performance and flexibility of WHDs. The vulnerability of wearable sensors is a significant issue that must be sensibly inspected. The usage of nanomaterial-based signal intensification is a possible improvement. Biostability must be carefully considered so that the sensors are covered by anti-microbial defensive coverings, stopping the possible contamination of nano-materials.

Advanced sensor supervision is taking place because wearable fitness plans can track many energetic signs in the human body. Everything is being monitored on a specific medium, from tracking infant's breathing to fitness requests or even the military on the battlefield. There are many opportunities to create great excitement in the WHDs.

REFERENCES

1. Ashton, K. "That 'internet of things' thing," *RFID Journal*, 22(7), 2009, 97–114.
2. Gubbi, J., Buyya, R., Marusic, S., Palaniswami, M. "Internet of Things (IoT): A vision architectural elements, and future directions," *Future generation computer systems*, 29(7), 2013, 1645–1660.
3. Fernandez, F., Pallis, G.C. "Opportunities and challenges of the Internet of Things for healthcare: Systems engineering perspective," *International Conference on Wireless Mobile Communication and Healthcare*, 263–266.

4. Jersak, L.C., da Costa, A.C., Callegari, D.A. "A Systematic Review on Mobile Health Care" *Tech. Report 073*, Faculdade de Informática PUCRS – Brazil, May 2013.
5. Fong, E.-M., Chung, W.-Y. "Mobile cloud-computing-based healthcare service by noncontact ECG monitoring" *Sensors*, 13(12), Dec. 2013, 16451–16473.
6. Deshpande, U.U., Kulkarni, M.A. "Iot based real time ecg monitoring system using cypress wiced," *International Journal of Advanced Research in Electrical. Electronics and Instrumentation Engineering*, 6(2), 2017.
7. Deshpande, U.U., Kulkarni, V.R. "Wireless ECG monitoring system with remote data logging using PSoC and CyFi," *International Journal of Advanced Research in Electrical Electronics and Instrumentation Engineering*, 2(6), 2013, 2770–2778.
8. Rani, S.U., Ignations, A., Vyasa Hari, B., Balavishnu, V.J. "IoT patient health monitoring system." *Indian Journal of Health Research and Development*, 2017, 1330–1334.
9. Tastan, M. "IoT based wearable smart health monitoring system," *Celal Bayar University Journal of Science*, 2018, 343–350.
10. Misbahuddin, S., Zubairi, J.A., Alahdul, A.R., Malik, M.A. "IoT- based ambulatory vital signs data transfer system," *Hindawi Journal of Computer Networks and Comunications*, 2018, 8 pages.
11. Dias, D., Silva Cunha, J.P. "Wearable health devices-vital sign monitoring systems and technologies," *MDPI Journal*, 18(8), 2018, 2414.
12. Wu, T., Redoute, J.-M., Yuce, M. "A wearable, low-power, real-time ECG monitor for smart T-shirt and IoT healthcare applications," *Springer Nature Switzerland*, 2019, 165–173.

Unit 2

IoT-Based Systems for Healthcare Sector
AI and Smart Computing

3 Machine Learning and Deep Learning in IoT-Based Healthcare Support Systems

Chandan Kumar Malik
Department of Pharmaceutical Technology
Jadavpur University

Debanjan Chatterjee
Department of Natural Products
National Institute of Pharmaceutical Education
and Research

CONTENTS

Customized medicine or personalized medicine (PH) is a new approach to patient care aimed at changing the conventional health system. Advanced patient data gathers wearable IoT (the Internet of Things), sensor devices and mobile devices from electronic health records, web-based information and social media. The healthcare system uses machine learning, AI techniques to collect datasets of disease point identification and auto-management of patient compliance and clinical intervention. For the last few decades AI has been very useful towards each and every aspects of our lifestyle which leads many progress of humankind. The flooding of this internet era and the sickness epidemic that arrived with the monsoon season of digitalization is developing into a humanitarian disaster. Several new initiatives have been made, and success has

DOI: 10.1201/9781003146087-5

been noticed. Drug metabolism and toxicity studies have been shifted to the drug discovery process with the help of CADD (Computer Aided Drug Design) technologies. Artificial intelligence (AI) also can significantly contribute to predicting drug metabolism and toxicity. Machine-deep learning (ML/DL) approaches are especially useful in taking up the work in this area. ML/DL are commonly used to synchronize analytical and silico models simultaneously. The models cover multiple service applications and help patients' clinical decisions to support their wellbeing. These analyse the data obtained from sensors and other sources to detect patient behavioural trends and clinical conditions. These models, for example, evaluate information gathered to assess the progress and behaviours of the patient. Here we will mention the test dataset and the training dataset for the efforts made in understanding drug metabolism and toxicity using AI techniques and patients' compliance. Based on the user knowledge, the input feed, the training dataset could be generated. Everything depends upon the wrong knowledge input provided by the user set.

3.1   INTRODUCTION

Recently, healthcare has used information technology to deliver intelligent systems for accelerating diagnosis and health treatment. In different ways, these systems provide intelligent health monitoring and medical automation services, allowing visiting costs to be drastically reduced and the quality of patient care to be improved overall [1]. One of these is IoT, defined as a global network that communicates with machinery and computers. There is no need for human interaction in this system since it contains autonomous features controlled by devices [2].

Health issues now happen at a high pace. A system that includes several sensors to collect information about human body parameters is designed to introduce a change in sensor technology. It will be transmitted on an IoT website that can be easily retrieved online by non-professionals using AI and ML/DL. Experts plan to raise the figure to 10 billion dollars by 2020 and 22 billion dollars by 2025, with more than seven billion IoT devices connected today [3].

AI is an IT branch with evolving ideas, methods, algorithms and frameworks for human intellect emulation and expansion [4]. In the first AI surge, beginning in the 1960s, AI system's core strength was expert information engineering; domain experts built computer programs for knowledge of very narrow application domains [5]. The second generation was focused on ML methods. Those involved in conventional ML methods build features, and feature engineering involves essential human beings. Models lack representative capacity and can form decomposable abstractions that automatically disconnect complex variables while forming observed data [6]. Deep learning methods with the help of AI reduce this problem to a profound, layered model framework and neural networks. The advancement of DL is significantly catalysed by the present interface and revival of the neural networks [7].

Big data analysis through ML provides tremendous advantages in assimilating and analysing vast volumes of complex healthcare data. ML is an AI type that includes algorithmic methods that allow machines to interpret and integrate different types of data (such as demographic data, laboratory reports, imaging data and free text notes) into disease risk forecasts, diagnosis prognosis and adequate treatments[8]. Implementation of medical data requires numerous DL algorithms, including an artificial neural network (ANN), genetic algorithms, decision processing and vector support (PVS). The structural elements of ANN involve processing devices (nodes or neurons) that are connected to a variety of adjustable weights that enable signals to pass across the network simultaneously and consecutively [9]. In general, ANN can be divided into three layers of neurons: input (receives information), hidden (responsible for the retrieval of patterns, mostly internal processing) and output. A genetic algorithm (GA) is a technology for search optimization focused on genetics and natural selection principles [10]. The application of genetics has promising consequences for diverse medical specialities, such as radiology, cardiology, endocrinology, gynaecology, pulmonology, infectious diseases, neurology and other healthcare management [3]. The decision tree is a formalism for expressing certain mappings and consists of tests or attribute nodes connected to two or more sub-trees and leaves or class-labelled decision nodes that mean decision. It can be applied for reviewing the medical literature for executing a meta-analysis and on systematic decision analysis. SVM essentially serves as the linear separator between two data points in the multi-dimensional setting to distinguish two distinct types. SVM uses a very large number, task-independent, non-linear functionality [11].

Drug metabolism estimation has acquired tremendous importance in pharmaceutical science. Many therapeutic candidates that fail in clinical trials are excluded because of the unpredictable effects of human metabolism, including toxicity and undesirable pharmacokinetic profiles. ML methods were used to model interactions between a compound and its metabolic fate. Resources currently available for defining *in silico* metabolic networks are divided into three categories: (1) structure–activity relationships (SAR) based computational model, (2) "pattern" tissue or organ response databases to drugs obtained from high-performance trials, (3) metabolic pathways, genes and regulatory networks[12].

This section summarizes different aspects of drug metabolism and toxicity using a system biology approach. Then we discuss the computational approaches, before eventually addressing the possibilities that may be realized by greater convergence of experimental and computational approaches.

3.2 DRUG METABOLISM AND TOXICITY

The path from the molecular goal and early medicine into the clinic is challenging, with several obstacles to overcome before a viable clinical candidate is created. The body is a complex system in which a therapeutic agent is absorbed, distributed, metabolized and/or excreted in several stages (ADME) [13]. There are places where drugs are regularly delivered, either intravascular or extravascular. Drugs delivered through the extravascular path must be absorbed to enter the blood. No absorption step is required during intravascular delivery. Specific formulations are needed for each administration site/route [13]. The most useful pharmacokinetic parameter for defining the absorption process is bioavailability [14]. Distribution is a way of moving a drug from and into the blood, tissues or bodies of the body following uptake.

Endocytosis, diffusion, which is passive and active transport, may lead to drugs being delivered across membranes; passive diffusion does not need resources. To travel passively, bases and weak acids must be in their non-ionized state. On the other hand, active transport includes energy and protein for transportation. The cell membrane contains a protein that binds the molecule, simplifies it, and requires no energy comparable to passive diffusions to move the gradient downward (for example, sugar, amino acids, and certain drugs such as penicillin and furosemide morphine). Endocytosis is the incorporation of drugs into small droplets or particles [15].

The pharmacokinetics of a potential drug must be ensured during medication for their expected pharmacological actions. Metabolism usually ends the expected action of the drug, although the metabolites can in some cases also be pharmacologically active compounds. Drug metabolization enzymes (DMEs) are essential to the metabolism, degradation and/or detoxification of xenobiotics or exogens in the body. Most of the tissues and organs have different DMEs to mitigate the possible damage caused by these compounds [10]. Phase I is oxidization, reduction or hydrolysis for incorporating the reactive oxygen species; phase II, conjugation of different moieties; phase III, degradation of the xenobiotics and metabolites through the use of hepatocytic and intestinal transporters [16]. Phase 1 DMEs consist primarily of a superfamily of cytochrome P450 (CYP) located in the liver, gastrointestinal tract, lung and kidney in great numbers [13]. Phase II enzyme metabolization or conjugation consists of several enzyme superfamilies, including sulfotransferases, UDP-glucuronosyltransferase (UGTs), epoxide hydrolases (EPH), Glutathione S-transferases (GSTs) and N-acetyltransferases [17]. Phase III transports P-glycoprotein (P-gp), a protein related to multidrug resistance (MRP), and organic anion (OATP2) are both transporters of phase III and are found in tissues like such brain, nephrological systems and the hepatic system [15]. There may be possible effects on multiple metabolism and pharmacokinetics of multiple therapeutic agents when controlling gene expression from various transporters, Phase II DME and Phase III [13]. As prescriptions are given and enter the general circulation, the body stimulates several forms of eliminating the drug. Excretion is the mechanism used for producing, removing and moving from the body to the exterior drugs and metabolites. The main excretory organs are the kidneys and liver. Organ clearance relies on blood flow in the same organ and drug extraction ratio as illustrated in equation no 1.

$$CLorgan = \frac{Rate\,of\,elimination}{Plasma\,concentration} \tag{1}$$

or

$$CLorgan = Q * E$$

where Q is the blood supply of an organ (i.e., the flow rate through an organ); (i.e., the fraction of the drug in the blood extracted by that organ on each passage through the clearing organ, or extraction ratio, or the intrinsic ability of the eliminating organ to clear the drug). This ranges between 0 (no removal) and 1 (complete extraction) [7].

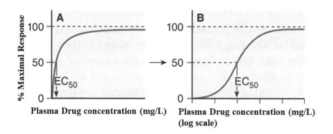

FIGURE 3.1 Graded response (y-axis as a percentage of maximum response) expressed according to drug concentration.

In pharmacodynamics, the relationship between the location of the drug accumulation and the period and severity of its adverse effects is described. The binding of the receiver determines the impact of a drug on the site. In the central nervous system (e.g., opioid receptor), neurons may have receptors for suppressing the feeling of pain, influence the heart muscle contraction if present on cardiac cells, or be responsible for maintaining bacterial cell wall integrity. The receptor region's concentration of medicine is correlated with pharmacological findings. Since the concentration logarithm is plotted against the effect, there is no effect below the concentration, and there is no greater effect over concentration: Figure 3.1 [18]. The effect and seriousness of drug reactions are the more marketed medicines. After intake, delivery, metabolism and excretion, various pharmaceuticals, herbal and medicinal reactions occur.

3.3   IN-SILICO DRUG METABOLISM AND TOXICITY

Before the in-silico modelling era, drugs were found by testing synthesized molecules using various in-vitro and in-vivo experiments. The candidate molecules investigate their pharmacokinetic properties, metabolization and possible toxicity in the further production of drugs. This technique allowed new leading compounds to be established. However, some promising lead compounds fail in the clinical process. That is why it is important to identify and stop the discovery route for weak drug candidates as soon as possible. The key reasons for stopping drug candidate production are weak pharmacokinetic properties and toxicity [19].

Therefore, solid screening technologies are increasingly important for providing early information on the properties of absorption, transmission, metabolism, excretion, and compound toxicity (ADME-Tox). Regulators were very concerned about in-silico or the estimation of pre-clinical toxicological endpoints, clinical adverse effects and ADME characteristics of new chemicals. The Food and Drug Administration (FDA) has used predictive toxicology software to support various regulatory testing criteria and initiatives [20]. Physiologically based simulations of pharmacokinetics (PBPK) incorporate both pharmacokinetic processes and drug-related data to model and simulate a pharmacokinetic drug profile in tissue and plasma. XenoSite is an important online server for predicting silico metabolism since it uses a neural network for modelling the Cytochrome P450 metabolism. For nine P450 isocyte servers, including 1A2, 2A6, 2B6, 2C8, 2C9, 2C19, 2D6, 2 E1 & 3A4, XenoSite is estimated

[21]. SMARTCyp 3.0 is a website metabolism predictor based on Python updated webserver for Cytochrome P450 mediated metabolism. The SMARTCyp programme is a concept based on Xenosite to detect the site of metabolism by measuring energy sources with more than 250 molecules using the theory of density function. New features include proximity calculations for the query molecule with the model fragment, a new graphical interface and additional configurations that enhance SMARTCyp structural coverage [22].

Molecular descriptors, using quantitative structure–activity relationship (QSAR), describe the relationship between molecules and their toxicity profile or other biological action in the case of drug toxicity studies [23]. In this modelling process, where the number of active compounds is far higher than the number of inactive compounds, the issue of imbalanced datasets is especially important. Binary models are calculated with confusion matrix values, in particular. True positive (TP), true negative (TN), false positive (FP) and false negatives (FN) are there. The sensitivity value is the model's ability to correctly predict positive (active) samples, while the specificity value is the model's ability to accurately predict negative (inactive) samples. The overall predictive power of the model is accurately measured (ACC).

$$\text{Sensitivity} = \frac{TP}{TP + FN}$$

$$\text{Specificity} = \frac{TN}{TP + FN}$$

$$\text{Balanced Accuracy} = \frac{Sensitivity + Sensitivity}{2}$$

Extensions of the classical model of QSAR are DEREK (deductive risk calculation from current knowledge) and TOPKAT (toxicity prediction by computer-assisted technology) [24]. DEREK is based on various laws made up of molecular substructure (structural alerts) concepts appropriate for toxic purposes (e.g., mutagenicity, cancer and/or inflammation of the skin). The regulations are not limited to chemical products. Still, they are used to generalize chemicals as subtraction is possible in many molecular environments (e.g. alkylating agent, acid or halogen-containing molecule) [25]. On the other hand, TOPKAT tests the composition properties of electrical topology (E-state) on any two possible atomic fragments, E-state atomic modification size calculated by a rescaled electron value count, molecular weight, symmetry index and topology shape [16]. To predict toxicity, Cramer suggested three structural groups. Class I includes essential chemistry substances and efficient metabolism methods suggesting low oral toxicity (e.g., compounds of the body (excluding hormones), HAA (Acyclic aliphatic hydrocarbons), Common terpenes, etc.). Class II compounds consist of substances with less harmful properties than Class I compounds. Still, they have no toxic structural characteristics, such as Class III compounds (e.g., alcohol, aldehyde, side-chain ketone, acid, ester, a bicyclic substance with or without a ring ketone etc.). Finally, Class III compounds, which are chemically arranged compounds, cannot be considered a simple initial defence or may even suggest significant toxicity or reactivate the functional group. This class contains structures that contain elements other than carbon or hydrogen, oxygen, nitrogen or divalent sulphur, some derivatives of benzene, some heterocyclic compounds [14].

3.4 ARTIFICIAL INTELLIGENCE AND DRUG DISCOVERY

Medical chemistry and especially "drug design" were sometimes perceived as more artistic, just like science. The market is considered time-consuming, hard, very expensive and a failure in clinical trial can create problem for that new drug candidate which is in the clinical trial final phase. The complexity of human disease has been argued for associated uncertainty regarding how to intervene in medical treatment and decision-making. More science will greatly support chemistry in the design and discovery of medicines. The development of computer algorithms can help a medicinal chemist. Here is a summary of the last two decades: examples of molecular automated de novo design, concepts and computers involve approaches and dare to anticipate several drug design options and limitations of intelligence with machines [26].

De novo design aims to create new (formerly unfamiliar) chemical entities from scratch with desired properties (i.e., pharmacological activity). There are three of these design concepts: (1) generation of molecules, (2) scoring of molecules, and (3) optimization of molecules. These are all separate or collective aspects that can be performed – by people or machines based on AI-learning methods [27]. Often in a few reaction steps, designs can be easily synthesized. In pharmaceutical industry the first fully automated synthesis and design of novel molecules in the lab was main challenges as manual intervention was there in each step .

A broad range of known bioactive compounds was included in simplified molecular-input line-entry (SMILES) to capture the repetitive neural network. Retinoid X has been refined in this general model, and peroxisome activated receptor agonists with proliferator activation through learning transfer. Five top-class molecules that were found to be effective in nanomolar concentration were designed by the model generative. The outcome of this study promotes artificial generative intelligence molecular design and demonstration prospective de novo the potential for future medicinal methods [28]

There is a training data model (i.e., molecular structures) that can be used in the field of exercise for the sampling of new cases (new chemical entities). There are several chemical entities with desired features. These generative methods should chemically produce correct structures without explicit requirements, including libraries of building blocks or fusion rules and chemical transformation (Figure 3.2). Only

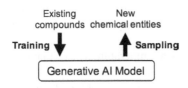

FIGURE 3.2 Genetic artificial intelligence (AI) definition.

retrospective de novo applied to AI design through reproduction or generation of known bioactive ligands actives forecast [11]. There were two basic computational approaches. First of all, a generic model was developed that learned the constitution of large, non-concentrated drug molecules compound sets. This generic has been improved in a second step model based on active library target-focused smaller molecular characteristics (SMILES).

The generic model using a deep recurrent neural network recently published long-term memory (LSTM) (RNN) cells which SMILES representations of 541,555 have been trained extracting bioactive compounds (KD, Ki, IC_{50} / EC_{50} < 1 mM). The compound database of ChEMBL22 was attached to a de novo target-specific ligands approach that was useful for producing 93% valid and 90% unique results. For example, 25 mimetic fatty acids with known purpose Retinoid X (RXR) agonistic activity and/or Peroxisome proliferator-activated receptor (PPAR) peroxisome receptors were chosen. They sampled 1000 SMILES for the resulting fine-tuned AI model application of fragment from the minimalist strings start fragment "Towards COOH functionalities." SMILES input, all carboxylic acid included as default function and the chemical structures of the compounds were identical sets of workouts. The newly produced molecules are important in populate training data chemical space, live in the fine-tuning set in the RXR/ PPAR region. These observations confirm the generative ability AI model to produce new chemical entities domain training [29].

3.5   HARDWARE REQUIREMENTS IOT

Health systems landscape, public health systems, health research, professional education systems and systems with many lacunae are fragmented; thus, the IoT platform has been launched. More advanced health data management and informative knowledge are needed based on expertise in computer public health. Platform technology is a new and highly integrated computer technology, combining internet technologies, websites, cloud, social technologies, and mobile applications. The public health approach provides an online infrastructure that enables more work synergies within each and all these systems. Professional health programmes need to be updated to understand profoundly and critically how platform technology should become the health sector foundation [30]. IoT-based hardware was designed and built for supporting health surveillance systems in popular circumstances, one of which is the ESP8266 Node MCU healthcare system. This system consists of MCU nodes, heartbeat sensor, cloud sensor, IoT, PLC, Thinger.io and mobile. MCU Node panels collect and transmit temperature and heartbeat sensor data in wireless mode. The dataset collected from different patients can be connected with a statistical package for the social science (SPSS) programme. It will help in future calculation and linear progression of data. The mobile health system, therefore, helps know people's real-time health conditions [31].

A digital thermometer is a temperature sensor that delivers 9° temperature measurement bits to 12 bits °C. The sensor can directly draw power from the data line with 3V to 5.5V voltage per unit. A single ROM board having a unique 64-bit serial code could measure in a temperature range of 55°C to +125°C or 67F to +257F) with + or – 0.5°C precision in the range +85°C -10°C [32].

The heartbeat sensor is based on photoplethysmography. It tests the changes in blood flow by any organ that induces a difference in light intensity by that regular body voltage. The instrument parts include ITR9904 diode emitting IR light as a photodiode and transmitter. The IR LED transmission is infrared placed on the fingertip, and then device ITR9904 can obtain the signal from the blood within the arteries by a photodiode. It can calculate the heart rate by measuring blood flow. The device is equipped with two low pass philtres with 100 gains each. This gain is sufficient to turn the weak signal into the signal of the heartbeat. LM358 circuit can be a heartbeat sensor that measures the heart rate of the pulse to 140.4 BPM with a frequency range of 2.34Hz. The heart rate can vary depending on how much the body needs during oxygen absorption, and carbon dioxide changes sleep or exercise [33].

The website Thinger.io is a Things Internet open-source platform. It is ready to link material with cloud infrastructure. The application is used to monitor the heartbeat and temperature at any point in time. SPSS is frequently used in research of health, marketing and education. SPSS analyses data for statistics descriptive and bivariate, numerical results identifying group forecasts [31].

A new C4.5 wrapper-based algorithm is proposed to help sound medical and health decision-making. The new S-C4.5-SMOTE sampling method can, in particular, address not only data distortion but also enhance the overall system output because its mechanism aims to efficiently reduce data size while preserving balanced and technically smooth datasets without distorting them. This achievement supports the wrapper approach of efficient selection without taking into account the issue of large volumes of data [31]: Figure 3.3.

Industry 4.0 covers many engineering and industrial management problems, such as development technology, new automation and data sharing [34], [35]. Concerning the technological Centre of Industry 4.0, it emphasizes the efficient implementation and incorporation of intelligent entities IoT, internet of services and cyber-physical systems (CPS) technology [36]. To promote the IoT industry 4.0, IoT has successfully been employed in various fields as "intelligence" plays a key role. Its wide range of applications covers transport and logistics, healthcare, intelligent environments (home, office, plant, etc.); its application is more prevalent in medicine and healthcare than in other fields. Furthermore, the development of RFID is one of the main technologies that promote more effective communication of IoT, in particular with passive RFID [37], [34], [27]. IoT is called the "Medical Internet of Things" (MIoT) when used for medical healthcare. MIoT aims to use intelligence-oriented IoT to link people, patients, medical personnel, drugs, different medical equipment and facilities to enable the automated identification, positioning, acquisition, monitoring, management and sharing of medical information. Smart primary IoT technology consists of (1) medical instruments and medicinal supplies, (2) digital clinics, and (3) remote medical treatment. In other words, MIoT aims to address medical and other questions [31]. The intelligent IoT service platform has successfully managed health issues. Remote health conditions have begun to generate enormous raw data,

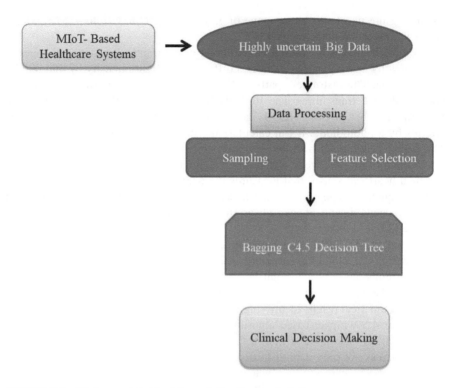

FIGURE 3.3   High uncertain big data analytics diagram in IoT.

mainly from IoT mobile healthcare systems, particularly due to the rapid growth of IoT technology. However, healthcare via mobile equipment used by people at home or in public is normally used to observe the appropriate health conditions or collect medical information. The raw data produced for clinical analysis and prediction can be further processed. The analysis of MIoT-based large data is helpful to facilitate both medical pre-diagnosis and the complementary treatment of patients by the large generation of data from the IoT-based healthcare system.

Furthermore, MIoT-based data should be reliable, efficient, stable, continuous and confidential [5]. Based on MIoT healthcare, an effective and efficient study of long-term health figures for wise clinical decision-making in the future is a positive target this decade. A new C 4.5 algorithm was developed using wrapper function selection to facilitate wise medical and healthcare clinical decisions. Still, managing the multidimensionality and high volume of data produced in MIoT-based medical systems is becoming increasingly necessary. Figure 3.4 sets out the following order to describe the relevant background of the IoTs. The advantages of the proposed method are illustrated in simulation examples, which then compare the results with those of the other methods. In particular, its application for clinical choice based on the ECG dataset is further carried out by the validation of proposed methods and clinical decision-making. The methodology proposed could also help answer classification

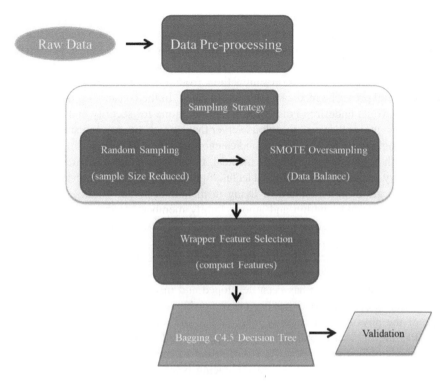

FIGURE 3.4 Data processing diagram process.

questions of 4.0 as regards functional implementation in real-life contexts, such as industrial engineering and management [31].

3.6 IOT IN HEALTHCARE SERVICES

IoT is a massively distributed, heterogeneous system that serves the needs of individuals and organizations. Today, mobile devices and contact systems are having an increasing effect on healthcare staff, consumers and the health industry. The range of wearable IoT-based products, instruments and apps is used in numerous surveillance applications to avoid death in hospitals or any other related area [38]. For enhanced health control and the control of inadequate medicines such as blood pressure (BP), haemoglobin (Hb), blood sugar, etc., a cooperative system of IoT is applied [39]. The distinctive characteristic of the system is that it is not important to find the node and move the source data. It is an effective strategy for critical health applications such as constant tracking and human health parameters. It is the first step towards green IoT and achieves a 57% electricity saving. A modern healthcare structure has been proposed to offer intelligent, customized and inclusive clinical services to single elderly people living with chronic disease. It helps patients to stay at home to get better treatment.

In some cases, that would minimize costs. The architecture suggested encourages patients to access online health services continuously and remote monitoring and care. The architecture of cloud-based healthcare allows for tracking industrial IoT structures that label health data until it moves into the cloud [40]. They have been using electrocardiogram (ECG) examinations from a health practitioner to diagnose disorders and prescribe medications to avoid death. In the consumer programme, the customer avoids undesired noise from a mobile phone for security and verification. The ECG signal is then sent to a cloud server that extracts time and spectrum features using a single-class SVM classifier and categorizes them [41].

E-health is an emerging field of medical, public and sector awareness. It affects the delivery of online healthcare and technological resources. IoT innovations enable patients to get a high standard of living in their own home. The role they recognize and settle down within and among family members decreases the burden on crowded healthcare facilities. IoT-enabled health networks only render home-health services workable by tracking the readings of the medical instruments to reduce the need for day-to-day medical visits. Public health interventions are analysed at three levels: public, personal and object [42].

The key index system has been developed and inspired the IoT side concept of healthcare. A modern model has been developed that involves the five-layered structure of the physiological sensing layer (PSL), the local connectivity layer (LCL), the IPL, the internet application layer (IAL) as well as the internet health service consumer application layer (UAL). According to the program model's definition, a complete network of motives for embracing healthcare was built with a literary review [43].

3.7 CONCLUSION

As an emerging media, the internet plays a crucial role in sharing knowledge. Through the exponential growth of internet-related networking technologies, the specifications for their further use are critical. Public health is critical in today's healthcare climate. IoT should be used as a social health structure. IoT is primarily a wireless internet communication platform that provides an in-house and outdoor approach to providing detailed knowledge of its surroundings and remotely controlling the environment. IoT provides various social and financial services and provides a high standard of quality and service. Education and healthy public policy must therefore be enforced. Therefore, creating and educating a proper community is essential for making e-health services usable with emerging technology accessible to citizens. Experimental metabolism techniques are subject to significant technical resources and human expertise demands.

This is where computer chemistry facilitates major advancements in metabolism research. Computational forecasts of drug metabolism are still a research file. This makes big progress in metabolism research easier for computational chemistry. Drug metabolism machine predictions are still an area of study. In-silico models, abortion, transmission, metabolism and excretion properties (ADME) of pharmaceutical molecules were expected. It needs both in vivo and in vitro simulated research trials to exclude non-significant variables from several factor parameters. The main task is to select and analyse the chosen model and reproduce it in real physiological environments. In parallel, implementing in-silico techniques improves forecasting toxic threats to humans and the climate. The data-driven models can be implemented to speed up decision-making by risk-screening, early detection and regulation of potential physicochemical toxicity and properties and optimize the use of knowledge that can also meet the manufacturing, regulatory and public requirements of safer chemicals. QSARs provide a research forum for assessing chemical toxicity with useful knowledge.

Currently, the pharmaceutical sector faces challenges in continuing its drug production owing to increased R&D expenses and reduced competitiveness. The task of finding effective potential products is daunting, the hardest aspect of drug development. The future applications of AI provide an ability to counteract the inefficiencies and contradictions in traditional approaches to drug manufacturing, eliminating bias and human intervention in the method. Experts believe that AI will forever transform the pharmaceutical business and how teaching algorithms and domain knowledge identify medicines. This creates an optimal working space where AI and medical chemists can collaborate very closely to evaluate vast databases and train devices, set algorithms or refine the evaluated data for a quicker and more reliable drug production method.

Depending on this AI, the hardware device made a major contribution in IoT-based healthcare, consisting of a temperature sensor, ECG module, GPS module, capacitors, etc. IoT is now considered a feasible solution for tracking solutions, particularly in fitness monitoring. It allows the securing of personal prosperity parameter data inside the cloud, decreasing hospital stays for conventional regular tests and, most significantly, the ability of every doctor to monitor wellbeing and disease diagnosis at a distance.

REFERENCES

1. Akmandor, Ayten O., Jha, Niraj K. "Smart Health Care: An Edge-Side Computing Perspective," *IEEE Consumer Electronics Magazine*, 7(1), 2017, 29–37.
2. Da Silva, Ivan Nunes, Spatti, Danilo Hernane, Flauzino, Rogerio Andrade, Bartocci, Luisa Helena Liboni, dos Reis Alves, Silas Franco. "Artificial Neural Network Architectures and Training Processes," *Artificial Neural Networks*, 2017, 21–28.
3. Matheny, Michael, Israni, Sonoo Thadaney, Ahmed, Mahnoor, Whicher, Danielle. "Artificial Intelligence in Health Care: The Hope, the Hype, the Promise, the Peril," *Natl. Acad. Med.*, 2020, 94–97.
4. Janardhanan, Padmavathi, Sabika, Fathima. "Effectiveness of Support Vector Machines in Medical Data Mining," *Journal of Communications Software and Systems*, 11(1), 2015, 25–30.
5. Kazmi, Sayada Reemsha, Jun, Ren, Yu, Myeong-Sang, Jung, Chanjin, Na, Dokyun. "*In Silico* Approaches and Tools for the Prediction of Drug Metabolism and Fate: A Review," *Computers in Biology and Medicine*, 106, 2019, 54–64.
6. Raies, Arwa B., Bajic, Vladimir B. "*In Silico* Toxicology: Computational Methods for the Prediction of Chemical Toxicity," *Wiley Interdisciplinary Reviews: Computational Molecular Science*, 6(2), 2016, 147–172.

7. Benedetti, Margherita Strolin, Whomsley, Rhys, Poggesi, Italo, Cawello, Willi, Mathy, François-Xavier, Delporte, Marie-Laure, Papeleu, Peggy, Watelet, Jean-Baptiste. "Drug Metabolism and Pharmacokinetics," *Drug Metabolism Reviews*, 41(3), 2009, 344–390.

8. Garrido, María J., Valle, Marta, Calvo, Rosario, Trocóniz, Iñaki F. "Altered Plasma and Brain Disposition and Pharmacodynamics of Methadone in Abstinent Rats," *Journal of Pharmacology and Experimental Therapeutics* 288(1), 1999, 179–187.

9. Lin, Tzong-Shyan, Liu, Pei-Yu, Lin, Chun-Cheng. "Home Healthcare Matching Service System Using the Internet of Things," *Mobile Networks and Applications*, 24(3), 2019, 736–747.

10. Meyer, Urs A. "Overview of Enzymes of Drug Metabolism," *Journal of Pharmacokinetics and Biopharmaceutics*, 24(5), 1996, 449–459.

11. Xu, Jun, Hagler, Arnold. "Chemoinformatics and Drug Discovery," *Molecules*, 7(8), 2002, 566–600, doi:10.3390/70800566.

12. Ray, Partha Pratim. "A Survey on Internet of Things Architectures," *Journal of King Saud University-Computer and Information Sciences*, 30(3), 2018, 291–319.

13. Simpson, Annemarie Elizabeth Claire Merryman. "The Cytochrome P450 4 (CYP4) Family," *General Pharmacology: The Vascular System*, 28(3), 1997, 351–359.

14. Hossain, M. Shamim, Muhammad, Ghulam. "Cloud-Assisted Industrial Internet of Things (Iiot)–enabled Framework for Health Monitoring," *Computer Networks*, 101, 2016, 192–202.

15. Kerb, Reinhold, Hoffmeyer, Sven, Brinkmann, Ulrich. "ABC Drug Transporters: Hereditary Polymorphisms and Pharmacological Impact in MDR1, MRP1 and MRP2," *Pharmacogenomics*, 2(1), 2001, *Future Medicine*, 51–64.

16. Xu, Changjiang, Yong-Tao Li, Christina, Kong, Ah-Ng Tony. "Induction of Phase I, II and III Drug Metabolism/transport by Xenobiotics," *Archives of Pharmacal Research*, 28(3), 2005, 249.

17. Hinson, Jack A., Forkert, Poh-Gek. "Phase II Enzymes and Bioactivation," *Canadian Journal of Physiology and Pharmacology*, 73(10), 1995, 1407–1413.

18. Andes, D., Craig. W.A. "Animal Model Pharmacokinetics and Pharmacodynamics: A Critical Review," *International Journal of Antimicrobial Agents*, 19(4), 2002, 261–268.

19. Alqahtani, Saeed. "In Silico ADME-Tox Modeling: Progress and Prospects," *Expert Opinion on Drug Metabolism & Toxicology*, 13(11), 2017, 1147–1158.

20. Yang, Chihae, Valerio Jr, Luis G., Arvidson, Kirk B. "Computational Toxicology Approaches at the US Food and Drug Administration," *Alternatives to Laboratory Animals*, 37 (5), 2009, 523–531.

21. Matlock, Matthew K., Hughes, Tyler B., Swamidass, S. Joshua. "XenoSite Server: A Web-Available Site of Metabolism Prediction Tool," *Bioinformatics*, 31(7), 2015, 1136–37.

22. Zaretzki, Jed, Matlock, Matthew, Swamidass, S. Joshua. "XenoSite: AccuratelyPredicting CYP-Mediated Sites of Metabolism with Neural Networks," *Journal of Chemical Information and Modeling*, 53(12), 2013, 3373–3383.

23. Lapenna, Silvia, Worth, Andrew. "Analysis of the Cramer Classification Scheme for Oral Systemic Toxicity-Implications for Its Implementation in Toxtree," *JRC Scientific and Technical Report EUR*, 2011, 24898.

24. Usak, Muhammet, Kubiatko, Milan, Shabbir, Muhammad Salman, Dudnik, Olesya Viktorovna, Jermsittiparsert, Kittisak, Rajabion, Lila. "Health Care Service Delivery Based on the Internet of Things: A Systematic and Comprehensive Study," *International Journal of Communication Systems*, 33(2), 2020, e4179.

25. Rohokale, Vandana Milind, Prasad, Neeli Rashmi, Prasad, Ramjee. "A Cooperative Internet of Things (IoT) for Rural Healthcare Monitoring and Control," In *2011 2nd International Conference on Wireless Communication, Vehicular Technology, Information Theory and Aerospace & Electronic Systems Technology (Wireless VITAE)*, 2011, 1–6.

26. Muster, Wolfgang, Breidenbach, Alexander, Fischer, Holger, Kirchner, Stephan, Müller, Lutz, Pähler, Axel. "Computational Toxicology in Drug Development," *Drug Discovery Today*, 13(7–8), 2008, 303–310, doi:10.1016/j.drudis.2007.12.007.

27. Hessler, Gerhard, Baringhaus, Karl Heinz. "Artificial Intelligence in Drug Design," *Molecules*, 23(10), 2018, doi:10.3390/molecules23102520.

28. Wu, Yunyi, Wang, Guanyu. "Machine Learning Based Toxicity Prediction: From Chemical Structural Description to Transcriptome Analysis," *International Journal of Molecular Sciences*, 19(8), 2018, doi:10.3390/ijms19082358.

29. Rydberg, Patrik, Gloriam, David E., Zaretzki, Jed, Breneman, Curt, Olsen, Lars. "SMARTCyp: A 2D Method for Prediction of Cytochrome P450-Mediated Drug Metabolism," *ACS Medicinal Chemistry Letters*, 1(3), 2010, 96–100, doi:10.1021/ml100016x.

30. Su Hlaing Phyo, Latt, Kyaw Zin. "Analysis on Healthcare System Using IoT," *International Journal of Trend in Scientific Research and Development (Ijtsrd)*, 3(4), 2019, 1336–1339, doi: https://doi.org/10.31142/ijtsrd25140.

31. Lee, Shin Jye, Xu, Zhaozhao, Li, Tong, Yang, Yun. "A Novel Bagging C4.5 Algorithm Based on Wrapper Feature Selection for Supporting Wise Clinical Decision Making," *Journal of Biomedical Informatics*, 78, 2018, 144–155. doi:10.1016/j.jbi.2017.11.005.

32. Gray, Kathleen. "Public Health Platforms: An Emerging Informatics Approach to Health Professional Learning and Development," *Journal of Public Health Research*, 5(1), 2016, 10–13. doi:10.4081/jphr.2016.665.

33. Onakpoya, Igho J., Heneghan, Carl J., Aronson, Jeffrey K.. "Worldwide Withdrawal of Medicinal Products because of Adverse Drug Reactions: A Systematic Review and Analysis," *Critical Reviews in Toxicology*, 46(6), 2016, 477–489, doi:10.3109/10408444.2016.1149452.

34. Helma, Christoph, Kazius, Jeroen. "Artificial Intelligence and Data Mining for Toxicity Prediction," *Current Computer Aided-Drug Design*, 2(2), 2006, 123–133. doi:10.2174/157340906777441717.

35. Basile, A.O., Yahi, Alexandre, Tatonetti, Nicholas P. "Artificial Intelligence for Drug Toxicity and Safety," *Trends in Pharmacological Sciences*, 40(9), 2019, 624–635, doi:10.1016/j.tips.2019.07.005.

36. Tatonetti, Nicholas P., Ye, Patrick P., Daneshjou, Roxana, Altman, Russ B. "Data-Driven Prediction of Drug Effects and Interactions," *Science Translational Medicine*, 4(125), 2012, doi:10.1126/scitranslmed.3003377.

37. Greco, Luca, Percannella, Gennaro, Ritrovato, Pierluigi, Tortorella, Francesco, Vento, Mario. "Trends in IoT Based Solutions for Health Care: Moving AI to the Edge," *Pattern Recognition Letters*, 2020.

38. Lei-hong, Liu, Huang Yue-shan, Wu Xiao-ming. "A Community Health Service Architecture Based on the Internet of Things on Health-Care," *World Congress on Medical Physics and Biomedical Engineering May 26–31, 2012, Beijing, China*, 2013, 1317–1320.

39. Deng, Li. "Artificial Intelligence in the Rising Wave of Deep Learning: The Historical Path and Future Outlook [Perspectives]," *IEEE Signal Processing Magazine*, 35(1), 2018, 177–180.

40. Jackson, Peter. *Introduction to Expert Systems.* 1998. Addison-Wesley Longman Publishing Co., Inc.
41. Murphy, Kevin P. *Machine Learning: A Probabilistic Perspective.* 2012. MIT Press.
42. Jiang, Fei, Yong Jiang, Hui Zhi, Yi Dong, Hao Li, Sufeng Ma, Yilong Wang, Qiang Dong, Haipeng Shen, Yongjun Wang. "Artificial Intelligence in Healthcare: Past, Present and Future," *Stroke and Vascular Neurology*, 2(4), 2017, 230–243.
43. Shahid, Nida, Rappon, Tim, Berta, Whitney. "Applications of Artificial Neural Networks in Health Care Organizational Decision-Making: A Scoping Review," *PloS One*, 14(2), 2019, e0212356.

4 An IoT-Based Smart Environment for Sustainable Healthcare Management Systems

M.N. Mohammed
Department of Engineering and Technology
Faculty of Information Sciences and Engineering
Management and Science University

Brainvendra Widi Dionova
Department of Electrical Engineering
Jakarta Global University

Salah Al-Zubaidi
Department of Automated Manufacturing Engineering
Al-Khwarizmi College of Engineering
University of Baghdad

Siti Humairah Kamarul Bahrain
Department of Engineering and Technology
Faculty of Information Sciences and Engineering
Management and Science University

Eddy Yusuf
Faculty of Pharmacy
Jakarta Global University

DOI: 10.1201/9781003146087-6

CONTENTS

Reliable safety systems are becoming increasingly necessary in cities worldwide. Although there is increasing improvement in technology, we have been required to pay attention to our lived environments. Indoor air quality (IAQ) is one of the most critical issues as ordinary people spend 90% of their time in a closed environment. Many health problems are caused by inhaling air pollution. Several investigations have been done on monitoring and controlling IAQ using Internet of Things (IoT) technology and how to reduce indoor air pollution that affects human health. In this chapter, the essential findings in the literature up to now in this evolving field have been reviewed, particularly the experimental details and the advantages of the various types of IAQ monitoring and controlling based on IoT systems that have been proposed. Moreover, the significant prospects for IoT technology are highlighted along with the future directions for further research in IAQ systems.

4.1 INTRODUCTION

Environmental quality is a set of characteristics of the environment as they impact human beings and other organisms. Environmental quality decay is one of the leading causes of civilization diseases. Air, water and soil are important elements of the environment that need intensive care because these elements are very important for human viability. According to the World Health Organization (WHO), 91% of the world's population lives in places where air quality falls below WHO guideline limits, with 3.8 million deaths every year caused by household air pollution [1]. Thus, there is a need to maintain and improve the quality of the environment to acceptable levels [2].

Indoor air pollution, due to toxic materials and other harmful chemicals, greatly influences the quality of indoor air; it is ten times worse than the pollution of outdoor air. The contaminated areas enable potential pollutants to grow more than in open spaces. Statistics in developing countries suggest that the health effects of indoor air pollution are much greater outdoor ones. The solid fuels that pollute indoor air account for more than 3.5 million deaths and a global daily-adjusted life year (DALY) of 4.5% in 2010 [3]. The quality of indoor air of a building is a major determinant for each person's healthy life and wellbeing and the productivity and comfort of humans. The concept of the Internet of things (IoT) is concerned with connecting different kinds of objects, such as smart mobile, PC, and tablets, to the internet, providing a newfangled type of communication between objects and individuals and between things. Various monitoring and controlling gadgets can assist human beings. In addition, different wireless technologies assist the connection from remote locations to enhance home environment intelligence. An advanced IoT network can cater for human beings' need to connect with other issues. The IoT technology has been developed with an innovative idea and a big growth of smart homes to enhance the standards of life [4].

As a consequence of increasing personal time spent indoors and mounting evidence from investigations into the quality of indoor air that lowering air pollutants is improving health styles [5], this review aims to highlight and appraise such studies on major air pollution, human health effects and indoor air quality (IAQ) systems. Furthermore, it highlights the large prospect of IoT technology. There can be further research to develop a controlling and monitoring system for IAQ to detect and reduce indoor air pollution harmful to human health in homes and the environment.

4.2 AIR POLLUTION AND HUMAN HEALTH IMPACTS

Air pollution refers to all destructive impacts of any sources that participate in the atmosphere pollution or degrading of its ecosystem. Air pollution is a result of human interventions or natural issues. It involves various types of pollutants, such as solid, liquid and gas materials [6]. The main sites that are constantly exposed to pollution are homes, industry and transportation sectors [7]. Developments in the industrial sector are increasing every year in several large and developing countries. But the increase of industrial development causes some detriment. Various processes in factories – welding, copper smelting, loading, melting, slag pouring and casting stage processes – causes air pollution in the form of fumes, gas, radiant energy and other hazards [8]–[13]. The motor vehicle has become an essential in everyday life, with a significant proportion of the populace travelling regularly by car. Poisons are created by tobacco smoke, organic pressurized canned products and discharges from the wide assortment of interior materials (particularly in recently produced vehicles) involving soft and hard plastics, glues, paints and oils [5], [14]. Sometimes ambient pollution enters and gets stuck in the car. Public transport generates a greater level of pollution than cyclists and pedestrians [15], [16].

Household indoor air (IAP) pollution is considered a major cause of mortality and morbidity and a big danger factor for childhood respiratory and other severe diseases. There are three major air pollutants: benzene, nitrogen dioxide, and carbon monoxide produced from fossil fuels for cooking, and particulate matter, increasing when there are more people [17]–[19]. Despite several physical activities that may produce various pollutants in the environment, environmental air pollution is majorly affected by anthropogenic activities [20]. Each kind of air pollution can lead to different diseases detrimental to human health. According to Saad et al., there are four main air pollutants and another four thermal comfort that are harmful to human beings [21].

4.2.1 PARTICLE POLLUTANTS

Particulate pollutants/particulate matter (PM) is often found in the air in or near industrial areas; USEPA explains that particulate matter is an air pollution term used in describing the mixture of solid particles and liquid droplets [22]. PM is divided into three types: coarse particles (PM_2), fine particles ($PM_{2.5}$) and ultrafine particles ($PM_{0.1}$) [23]. PM varies in size from 2.5 to 10 μm. There are physical characteristics of the human respiratory effect because the size of the particle has been directly linked to being the main cause of health problems, namely respiratory mode, rate and volume [24]. Thus, PM can lead to premature death, chronic bronchitis, asthma attack, diabetes, cardiovascular disease and otherwise restrict activity [25].

4.2.2 GROUND-LEVEL OZONE

Ground-level ozone is one of the six major air pollutants and second-ranked of pollution that is harmful to human health [22]. Ozone (O_3) is colourless air pollution and can be found in the upper atmosphere (stratosphere). However, O_3 can also be found in the troposphere, which is not good for health [23]. If humans continually inhale ozone, it can cause permanent damage to the lungs, respiratory infection, reduce lung function, cause asthma, emphysema or bronchitis [26]. Besides having a negative impact on human respiratory health, O_3 also has an impact on skin health (two types of skin cancer – melanoma and non-melanoma), eyes (photokeratitis, blindness, cataract that causes by eye lens damaged by oxidative agents) and the human immune system (suppression of immune response to skin cancer, infectious diseases and other antigens) [27].

4.2.3 CARBON MONOXIDE

Carbon monoxide (CO) is an important criteria pollutant ubiquitous in an urban environment. CO is colourless, odourless and tasteless air pollution made from incomplete combustion of fuels, as in burning coal and wood [28]. CO is often found inside or outside the room, which can enter the circulation of the foetus and evolving brain through the placenta [29]. Poisoning by CO readily causes weakness, headache, nausea, vomiting, dizziness and loss of consciousness because the tendency of CO to haemoglobin is about 250 times greater than oxygen [6], [30].

4.2.4 SULPHUR DIOXIDE

SO_2 is a toxic, significantly reactive gas that is considered a noteworthy pollutant of air. It is primarily released from petroleum product utilization, customary volcanic activities, and factory operations. SO_2 is uncommonly pernicious for the wellbeing of humans, animals and plant life. The lungs and skin of individuals who are constantly subjected to such gas are susceptible to infection. The important health issues associated with high exposure to SO_2 include breathing disturbance and exacerbation of existing cardiovascular illness. SO_2 predominantly affects the upper airways. As a material irritation, it can create bronchospasm and real liquid emanation in individuals. Occupants of industrial areas who are exposed to even a low amount of SO_2 (<1 ppm) of polluted air may encounter an elevated level of bronchitis [6].

4.2.5 NITROGEN DIOXIDE

Nitrogen Dioxide (NO_2) is air pollution that is usually generated from motor engines. NO_2 is not as dangerous as ozone, but inhaling this pollution with a 2.0–5.0 ppm concentration may cause T-lymphocytes [6]. NO_2 can also cause respiratory infections such as bronchial reactivity, aggravation of chronic respiratory and asthma diseases [31]. Children affected by inhaling NO_2 gas can increase their exposure to respiratory illnesses such as pneumonia, asthma and other lower respiratory infections [32].

4.2.6 VOLATILE ORGANIC COMPOUNDS

Volatile Organic materials (VOCs) are a crucial class of indoor air pollutants. Many investigations and studies have revealed that building material and furnishings form 60% of VOCs indoor emissions [33]. The sources of VOCs emissions come from cleaning products, furniture and artistic products, including formaldehyde, benzene or toluene [34]. In addition to the harmful impacts of many VOCs, it was shown that VOCs cause asthma and asthma-associated symptoms [35]. Besides asthma, other diseases caused by inhaling VOC are respiratory diseases, anaphylactic diseases, cardiovascular diseases and cancer [36].

4.2.7 TEMPERATURE

The temperature in a room used for all kinds of activities does not have a threshold point, but for the best working environment the best temperature is around 20–24°C [37]. Poor air temperature control can impact performance implicitly through its effect on the predominance of Sick Building Syndrome (SBS) indications or fulfilment with air quality. Slowing down the learning effect, warm discomfort is affected by poor temperature quality [38]. Eyestrain, perspiration, accelerated respiration, dizziness, and heart rate are sensitive self-reported symptoms that the human body responds to with gradual temperature changes [39].

4.2.8 Humidity

The relative humidity of air is the water content ratio contained in the air at a specific temperature [37]. Relative humidity changes daily and (often) seasonally, and the utilization of average relative humidity does not represent the mean moisture content of the air [40]. Low humidity causes many issues like dry and irritated eyes and flaky and itchy skin and dries out and inflames the mucous membrane lining the respiratory tract [41]. In addition, humidity can influence microbial pollutants indoors and increase heart disease admissions [42], [43].

4.2.9 Indoor Air Quality

The purpose of monitoring IAQ is to understand the effect on human health, comfort and wellbeing within and around occupied buildings and structures [44]. Figure 4.1 shows daily human time activity allocation. IAQ is a critical problem because humans spend approximately 90% of their time breathing "indoor air" (at home, work or school). In contrast to open air, indoor air is reused constantly, making it trap and develop poisons. IAQ affects the percentages of toxins for indoor air, as does air temperature and relative humidity [45].

The increased societal patterns of population densification, work and family structure, childcare dependence, the purchase and use of items, including motor vehicles, that contribute to indoor air pollution, have raised the risk of spreading airborne infection [7]. As a result, poor IAQ is caused by pollution generated from inside the room and air pollution coming from outside the room, poor cleaning practices, poor moisture control, human occupancy, and poor building maintenance. To improve IAQ, a cleaning and vacuuming machine can be used to improve air circulation inside and outside the room and otherwise [37].

4.3 IOT ARCHITECTURE OF IAQ

Since IoT associates everything and everybody to trade data among themselves, the traffic and stockpiles in the system will likewise increase in exponential behaviour.

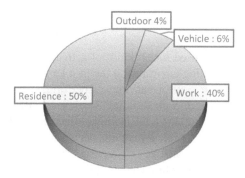

FIGURE 4.1   Daily human time activity allocation [45].

Hence, IoT advancement relies upon innovation and new applications and business activities [46]. Three layers have been defined, namely, the sensing, network and the application layers. ZigBee and Wi-Fi are utilized for communicating all those three layers. However, any other related technology can be adopted for this purpose. According to the edge-computing mechanism, the balancing and distribution of the total workload can be performed over these three layers [47], [48].

4.3.1 Sensing/Perception Layer

This layer is considered as the basis of the whole monitoring system. It is mainly responsible for air quality sensing. The nodes of sensing represent the major elements of the sensing layer, which can be deployed along the large zone. The details of the hardware and software of these nodes will be presented in the next section. Contingent upon the kinds of sensors, the data can be: temperature, area, movement, direction, vibration, speed, humidity, noticeable chemical alters and so on. The gathered data is then delivered to the network layer for its protected transmission to the data processing framework. Sensor systems can be used for smart building environmental data (temperature and moistness, and so forth.), construction hardware, heating, ventilation and air conditioning systems, plumbing, power control and distribution systems, lighting and different subsystems. These acquire constant data in real time in different frameworks through sensors and send to smart structures or control centres [46], [47], [49]. The examples of sensing/perception sensors, such as gas sensors (MQ-131, MQ-135, and MQ-7), particulate matter sensors (DSM501a) and temperature and humidity sensors (DHT11/DHT22), are shown in Table 4.1.

4.3.2 Networking/Edge-Computing Layer

Edge-computing devices (ECDs, IoT gateways) are the elements of this layer. Their function is to communicate and interact with the other two layers. First, ECDs collect the required data from the sensing layer to pass this data later to the application layer. The transmission media can be wireless or wired, while technology may be UMTS, 3G, Wi-Fi, infrared, ZigBee, Bluetooth, etc., relying upon the sensor gadgets [46], [47]. Table 4.2 explains the characteristics and standards of connectivity using ZigBee, Wi-Fi, Thread, Bluetooth LE and Z-Wave. The characteristic of this wireless network helps to determine the level of connectivity that suits some tasks.

4.3.3 Application Layer

The application layer is mindful of collaborating services to the clients and information storage. It is classified into two segments, namely, IoT cloud (IBM cloud) and user applications. Once it gets the recorded data from the ECD, it saves the information within the cloud database, giving visualized information in various ways. The applications executed by IoT can be intelligent wellbeing, smart cultivating, intelligent home, smart city, smart transportation, and so forth [46], [47]. The layers of IoT architecture of the monitoring system are shown in Figure 4.2.

TABLE 4.1
Air Pollution Sensor

S. No.	Hardware	Type of Sensor	Air Pollution
1.		MQ-7 [50]	CO
2.		MQ-135 [51]	NH3, NOx, Alcohol, Benzene, Smoke, CO_2
3.		MQ-131 [52]	Ozone, CL_2, NO_2
4.		MQ-2 [53]	Methane, Propane, Hydrogen, Alcohol, Liquefied Petroleum Gas
5.		DHT11 [54]	Temperature, Humidity
6.		DSM501a [53]	Particulate matter

TABLE 4.2
Characteristics of Network Wireless [55]

Characteristics	ZigBee	Wi-Fi	Thread	Z-wave	Bluetooth LE
IEEE standards	802.15.4	802.11	802.15.4	N/A	802.15.1
Frequency band	2.4GHz	2.4 GHz, 5GHz	2.5 GHz	900 MHz	2.4 GHz
Standard range	100m	150 m	30 m	30 m	10 m
consumption of Peak current	30 mA	116 mA	12.3 mA	17 mA	12.5 mA
consumption of Power per bit	185.9 µW/bit	0.000525 µW/bit	117 µW/bit	0.71 µW/bit	0.153 µW/bit
Rate of Data	250 Kbps	1Gbps	250Kbps	100Kbps	1Mbps
Network configuration	Star, Cluster, Mesh	Star, Mesh	Mesh	Mesh	Star, Bus
Nodes Number per network	65000	250/access point	300	232	One to many

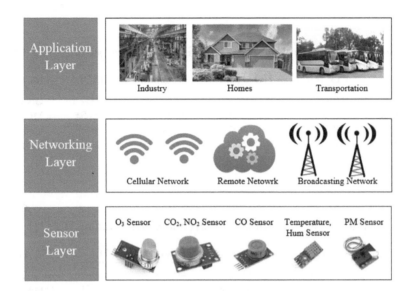

FIGURE 4.2 Architecture of IoT IAQ System [48].

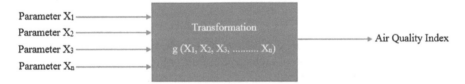

FIGURE 4.3 Air quality index calculation [56].

4.4 INDOOR AIR QUALITY INDEX

The term "air quality index" is a schema able to convert the weighted air values of pollution factors (for instance, the concentration of CO or visibility) into a unified value or group of numbers [56]. Hence, the air quality index is used as a key tool to understand pollution. Consequently, air quality indicators are used to standardize and collect air pollutant data and allow comparisons to be promptly attempted and fulfil public requests for precise, simple to interpret information. Furthermore, the user is provided with the required knowledge by the air quality indicators for tracking air status to eliminate the need to understand the comprehensive monitoring data [57]. Figure 4.3 shows the air quality index calculation block that contains n air parameters and transforms them into the air quality index.

The IAQ index (IAQI) describes the level of indoor air pollution and related health impacts. The IAQI is limited to the health effects on humans during exposure to unhealthy air for a few hours or days. Table 4.3 and Table 4.4 are the standards acceptable for indoor air pollution and other pollutants from IAQ and thermal comfort. The two indexes (i.e. IAQI and TCI (thermal comfort index)) are classified into

TABLE 4.3
The Threshold Ranges of Indoor Air Pollution and Corresponding IAQI [21]

CO_2 (ppm)	CO (ppm)	NO_2 (ppm)	O_3 (ppm)	IAQI	IAQI status
340–600	0.0–1.7	0–0.021	0–0.025	100–76	Good
601–1000	1.8–8.7	0.022–0.08	0.026–0.05	75–51	Moderate
1001–1500	8.8–10	0.09–0.17	0.051–0.075	50–26	Unhealthy
1501–5000	10.1–50	0.18–5	0.076–0.1	25–0	Hazardous

TABLE 4.4
The Threshold Ranges of Thermal Comfort and Corresponding TCI [21]

PM10 (gm/m³)	VOC (ppm)	Temp (0c)	Humid (%)	TCI	TCI status
0–0.02	0–0.087	20–26	40–70	100–76	Most Comfort
0.021–0.15	0.088–0.261	26.1–29	70–80	75–51	Comfort
0.151–0.18	0.262–0.43	29.1–39	80–90	50–26	Not Comfort
0.181–0.6	0.44–3	39.1–45	90–100	25–0	Least Comfort

four levels with different air pollution for each level. Each level of the air quality index has a range point (e.g. unhealthy/not comfortable 50–26), which is determined by detecting the concentration of eight types of air pollution and combining, calculating all parameters into one [58].

To achieve the environmental IAQ index (EIAQI), two independent indexes were created: IAQI and TCI[59]. After getting IAQ index (IAQI) weightage for each parameter of indoor air pollution and TCI other pollutants, IAQI and TCI weightage summing will be performed to obtain the EIAQI index. Each sub-index produces IAQI and TCI weightage for each level; after that, it will be classified according to the EIAQI level. For example, suppose the sum of air pollution and other pollutants has a total weightage point below one. It is categorized as the worst index, and the total weightage point is between 2–3, then the bad index is categorized, the total weightage point is 4–5. Finally, the good index and weightage point 6 are categorized as excellent [21]. The calculation procedure of the EIAQI is shown in Figure 4.4. The AQI may act as a solution; however, the AQI scales vary according to location as there are several air quality standards, and organizations may select various levels of classes that create an obstacle for a fair comparison and reduces its usability [60].

4.5 IAQ MONITORING AND CONTROLLING SYSTEM USING IOT TECHNOLOGY

IAQ monitoring is changing fast as miniaturized, cheap air sensors are enabling consumers, cities, community groups, and businesses. Air quality monitoring is a technique to give data about specific sorts of contamination levels. IAQ monitoring is

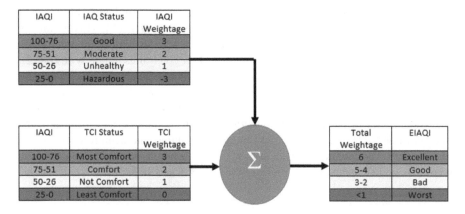

IAQI	IAQ Status	IAQI Weightage
100-76	Good	3
75-51	Moderate	2
50-26	Unhealthy	1
25-0	Hazardous	-3

IAQI	TCI Status	TCI Weightage
100-76	Most Comfort	3
75-51	Comfort	2
50-26	Not Comfort	1
25-0	Least Comfort	0

Σ

Total Weightage	EIAQI
6	Excellent
5-4	Good
3-2	Bad
<1	Worst

FIGURE 4.4 Calculation of environment IAQ index (EIAQI) [21].

typically via sensor-based devices. Part of them can estimate parts per billion levels and come as either mixed gas or portable units [61], [62].

In any case, since most systems monitoring air quality provide the detected numerical estimation of the corresponding toxin without change, it is hard for non-expert clients to determine how great air pollution is or determine the pollution criteria of every poison. Indeed, one of the significant tasks of an IoT-based monitoring system for air quality is to advise on the present air-quality status more instinctively and thoroughly progressively, instead of giving general clients individual numerical data regarding every poison. To accomplish this, it is essential for the system monitoring air quality to advise clients of the data about the present air quality utilizing an instinctive showcase device that can demonstrate air-quality level progressively [63].

The primary job of air investigation and checking is to acquire solid explanatory data concerning a few instruments and procedures. The first is to distinguish proof of poison emanation sources and appraisal of the scope of their impact. The subsequent one is the appraisal of the ecological quality and examining the natural destiny of pollutants. As of late, a few modern systems have been produced to track environmental status, consistently enhancing IAQ [2] effectively.

In response to indoor air pollution, a control system, using ventilation, is the most efficient method to enhance IAQ. Ventilation and shading can assist in the control of indoor temperatures. Ventilation also enables removing the indoor airborne pollutant that originally came from the indoor-based source. This minimizes pollutant levels and enhances IAQ. Careful evaluation of air circulation must be done to lower the level of polluted indoor air where pollutants outdoor sources may be available, like refuse and smoke [64,65].

4.6 APPLICATION OF IAQ MONITORING ON INDUSTRY, HOMES AND TRANSPORTATION

IAQ monitoring is changing fast as miniaturized, cheap air sensors are enabling consumers, cities, community groups, and businesses [66]. Online continuous monitoring is required nowadays for urban ecosystems due to the direct influence of air quality on health, productivity, safety, and people's prosperity [67], [68]. This monitoring system combines low and high specifications of gas sensors with serial communication to easily monitor and provide notification of air conditions remotely [69]–[72].

IoT and big data technology provide the data collection and show the information in real time. To synchronize with environmental alterations, the lives of its users are expected to be easier and more comfortable at that location. Thus, the utilization of IoT systems can be performed by integrating multi-module devices to retrieve data like Wi-Fi and RTC (real time clock) modules, Arduino microcontroller board and sensors [62]. The monitoring system of air quality on houses, vehicles and industry sectors using IoT technology is revealed in Table 4.5 and Table 4.6.

TABLE 4.5

Air Quality Monitoring Applications on Homes and Industry Using IoT Technology

S. No.	Title and Year	Pollutants	Sensors
1.	Air Quality Monitoring System Based on IoT using Raspberry Pi (2017)	Particulate Matter, CO, CO_2, Temperature, Relative Humidity, Pressure [73]	DHT22, DSM501a, MQ135, MQ9, BMP180
2.	Monitoring System of IoT Based Air Pollution (2019)	Temperature, Humidity, Smoke, LPG, CO, Particulate matter [74]	DHT11/DHT22, MQ2, SDS021
3.	The IoT Enabled Proactive Monitoring System of IAQ (2017)	Ozone [75]	MQ131
4.	IoT Enabled Real-Time Bolt based IAQ Monitoring System (2019)	Ammonia, Smoke, VOCs, Benzene [76]	MQ135
5.	IoT implementation of Kalman Filter air quality monitoring (2018)	Particulate matter, CO, NO_2, SO_2, O_3 [70]	ZH03A Laser, SGA-700
6.	Monitoring System of IOT Based Air Pollution (2018)	NH_3, NOx, Alcohol, Benzene, Smoke, CO_2, LPG, Temperature and Humidity [77]	MQ135, MQ6, LM35, SY-HS-220
7.	IoT-Enabled Air Quality Monitoring Device (2018)	Light, Gas, HCHO, Temperature [78]	Light, Gas, CO_2, HCHO, and Temperature sensors
8.	Wireless Sensor Network based on Raspberry Pi Air Pollution Monitoring (2017)	Temperature, Humidity, Gas, CO, Light [79]	DHT22, MQ135, MQ7, LDR,
9.	SPIRI: Low Power IoT Solution for Monitoring IAQ (2018)	Temperature, Humidity, Pressure, VOC, eqCO$_2$, Particulate matter, CO_2, Luminosity, Sound, Energy [71]	BME280, CCS811, PMS70031, CDM7160, TSL4531, SPH0645LM4H, Energy, PIR

(Continued)

TABLE 4.5 (Continued)
Air Quality Monitoring Applications on Homes and Industry Using IoT Technology

S. No.	Title and Year	Pollutants	Sensors
10.	A high precise E-nose for daily IAQ monitoring (2017)	Temperature, Humidity, H_2, CO, Ethanol, Ammonia, CH_4, Toluene [72]	SHT10, QS-01, TGS2600, TGS2602
11.	Air Quality Monitoring by Wireless Sensor Network (2018)	CO_2, NO_3, Temperature, Humidity [80]	MQ135, DHT22[80]
12.	Enabling of Wireless Sensing and Monitoring Air Quality by Customized IoT (2018)	Temperature, Humidity, Light [81]	SHT11, TSL2561
13.	IAQ Monitoring (2018)	Ozone, SO_2, NO_2, CO [82]	MQ2
14.	Air Pollution Detector System (2016)	CO [83]	MQ7
15.	IAQ Monitoring Using Wireless Sensor (2012)	CO, CO_2, Aerosols (PM2.5, PM10) [84]	TGS 2442, TGS 4161, Dust track DRX Aerosol 8533

TABLE 4.6
Air Quality Monitoring Applications on Transportation Vehicle Using IoT Technology

S. No.	Title and Year	Pollutants	Sensors
1.	Portable Electronic Nose (2012)	VOCs, Temperature, Humidity, Formaldehyde, Benzene, Toluene, CO, NO_2 [85]	GSBT11, TGS2620, TGS2602, O_2-A1, TGS2201, DHT22
2.	Carbon Monoxide Monitoring and Alert System for Automobiles (2013`)	CO [86]	MQ5
3.	Intelligent in-vehicle air quality management (2016)	PM2.5, TVOC [87]	In-vehicle air quality sensor
4.	Vehicle Cabin Air Quality Monitoring (2017)	CO, NO_2 [88]	TGS-2442, GLG-0710, MiCS-4512, $MoO3$-TiO_2
5.	MEMS Car Cabin Air Quality (2006)	VOC, Cigarette smoke, Fast food odour and manure, Bio effluents [89]	MEMS, Pd3, Pt02, U, temperature and humidity sensor
6.	CO Detection and Control Vehicle Cabin System (2015)	CO [90]	MQ7
7.	Real-Time Air Quality Monitoring in Metropolitan Area (2013)	Particulate Matter, CO [91]	Sharp dust sensor, MQ7

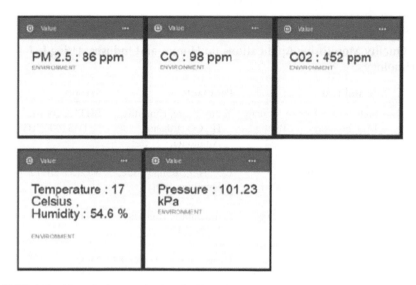

FIGURE 4.5 Air pollution monitoring dashboard [56].

Table 4.5 and Table 4.6 are examples of air quality monitoring application systems. These monitoring systems aim to detect air pollution such as CO, NO_2, PM, VOC, temperature and humidity inside a room by using a gas sensor (MQ sensor) and sending air pollution data to a mobile application that can be monitored easily by the user. Before air pollution data is sent to a mobile application, it is processed in a microcontroller to get air pollution conditions at this time (good, moderate and hazardous) [83]. Figure 4.5 shows an air pollution monitoring dashboard that contains six air pollution. Figure 4.6 shows the air quality index for each pollutant (PM10 and CO_2) and the real-time air pollution monitoring chart application dashboard. Figure 4.7 shows the AQI using a java application that contains AQI points, the most responsible pollutant in the room, the most dangerous room due to gas contamination and AQI based on colour code.

4.7 APPLICATION OF IAQ CONTROLLING SYSTEMS

Polluted indoor air has a harmful and risky impact on the environment and people's health. An IAQ controlling system is a technique employed to reduce or eliminate emissions or pollutants that can harm the environment or human health using ventilation systems (natural, mechanical and hybrid). Ventilation reduces indoor air pollution produced from humans, indoor activities and building materials [92].

The natural ventilation principle is to get maintainable utilization of environment normal inputs. This implies that the selected design method applies just from existing surrounding resources, such as wind, sunlight, and airflow, to acquire a thermally comfortable level to the indoor temperature [93]. The mechanical ventilation system is an air cleaner used to circulate air from outside into the room or otherwise by adding air pollution or temperature control before the air enters the room [92]. Hybrid ventilation is a combination of manual and mechanical ventilation systems that can

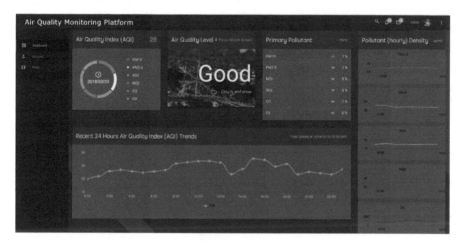

FIGURE 4.6 Air quality index monitoring application dashboard [70].

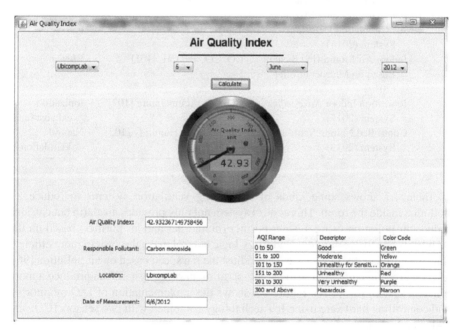

FIGURE 4.7 Air quality index monitoring system [84].

be alternated in the selection process. The purpose of hybrid ventilation systems is to minimize energy utilization and keep a satisfactory indoor status. Integrated ventilation systems are equipped with intelligent systems to control natural mode selection or mechanical ventilation (control by activating or deactivating a switch) [94]. Hence, the nominal pollutant must be recognized to minimize the steady-state concentration at or below an acceptable, comfortable and safe concentration level.

TABLE 4.7
Application of IAQ Controlling Systems

S. No.	Title and Year	Pollutants	Ventilation Systems
1.	Intelligent IAQ Monitoring and Purification Device (2017)	Aldehydes, Alcohols, Ketones, PM2.5, Temperature and Humidity [95]	Humidifier, air purifier
2.	IAQ Monitoring and Controlling (2019)	PM10, CO_2 [96]	Ventilation Fan
3.	Automated Control IAQ System (2017)	Temperature, Methane, CO, Propane and Smoke [97]	Water sprinkler, exhaust fan
4.	Carbon Monoxide Monitoring and Alert System for Vehicle (2019)	CO [98]	Power Window
5.	Carbon Monoxide and Total Suspended Particulate Ejector System (2018)	CO, TSP [99]	Ejector
6.	Air Circulation Detection System (2014)	Temperature, CO [100]	Fan
7.	Indoor Air Monitoring System Based on Microcontroller (2017)	CO, CO_2 and CH_4 [101]	Blower
8.	Ionization Indoor Air Purifier System (2015)	CO, CO_2, Temperature [102]	Ionization, exhaust fan
9.	Controlled Natural Ventilation System (2013)	Temperature, Humidity [103]	Natural Ventilation

Table 4.7 shows some kinds of controlling ventilation systems to reduce air pollution inside the room. This control system not only provides an alarm but can also reduce air pollution using a water purifier (humidifier and air purifier) based on the AQI [95]. The IoT technology and fuzzy logic control make the system more efficient than the normal system because it can adjust the fan speed based on air pollution [96]. IAQ controlling combined with an indoor air monitoring system can produce a more efficient system [5], [104]. Figure 4.8 shows the implementation of IAQ monitoring and controlling hardware using IoT technology combined with two sensors (CO_2 and PM_{10}) and a fan.

4.8 BENEFITS OF MONITORING AND CONTROLLING SYSTEMS OF IAQ USING IOT TECHNOLOGY

The monitoring and controlling system of IAQ that uses IoT technology is a powerful tool to analyse air quality and electrical consumption, support decision-making, and reduce indoor air pollution. The benefits of utilizing IAQ controlling and monitoring systems based on IoT technology are described below:

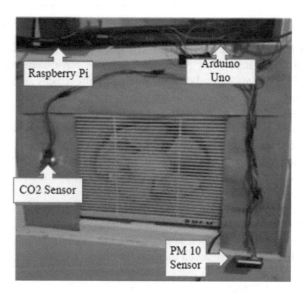

FIGURE 4.8 Indoor air circulation control using IoT technology [96].

- The air quality system is appropriate for online home safety monitoring and wireless controlling of home appliances and protection from fire accidents with immediate solutions [4].
- Air pollution monitoring integrated with mobile applications assists the client in estimating pollution and AQI levels. In addition, the application has some features such as indices of air quality using online estimation and air quality dips related to health risks [48].
- This air quality monitoring is very useful as the air quality can be monitored within the Android mobile system. It also alerts and generates notifications whenever the IAQ is reduced beyond the acceptable limit [76], [78].
- According to the ASHRAE standard, IoT and fuzzy logic-based systems for monitoring and controlling IAQ can maintain the quality index of indoor air (AQI) at an acceptable and safe level [96].
- The monitoring and controlling system can track the quality of indoor air progressively and effectively to ensure qualified air by utilizing an air purifier and humidifier [95].
- The CO detection systems have quick response and precise sensing of any basic or crisis state that deal with it directly and empower quicker dissemination of CO gases [98].
- This IAQ system is incredibly valuable in observing air quality status inside a building to more readily comprehend the present condition of air quality to consider the conduct of environmental conditions [105].
- A ventilation system can optimize air conditions such as IAQ and thermal comfort for individuals living or operating there, considering their health, prosperity and comfort [104].

4.9 CONCLUSION

IoT has been utilized in various sectors involving smart home, healthcare, automotive, and different industries. Several IoT devices have been combined in our daily lives. IoT integrates several devices supplied with sensing, identification, processing, communication, and networking capabilities. This research aims to know the effect on human health, comfort and wellbeing within and around occupant buildings and structures. This research summarizes major air pollution and various monitoring and controlling systems for the quality of indoor air using IoT technology. The monitoring and controlling of the IAQ play a crucial role in assisting human health, especially to give a real-time report, alert and reduce air pollution to improve the quality of life.

Most commonly, IAQ control systems do not use IoT technology. Developments in IAQ control systems facilitate the conducting and building of an integrated system controlled remotely. This research has presented the state of the art on air quality systems using IoT technology based on the IAQ index. This chapter can act as a significant starting point for future researchers to investigate the relationship between IAQ systems using IoT technology.

REFERENCES

1. WHO. *Ambient air pollution: A global assessment of exposure and burden of disease.* 2016. WHO.
2. Mar, M., Tobiszewski, M., De, M., Namie J. "Analytica Chimica Acta Current air quality analytics and monitoring: A review," 853, 2015, 116–126.
3. Kankaria, A., Nongkynrih B., Gupta, S.K. "Indoor air pollution in India: Implications on health and its control," 39, 2014, 203–208, https://doi.org/10.4103/0970-0218.143 019.
4. Pavithra, D., Balakrishnan, R. "IoT based monitoring and control system for home automation," *Glob Conf Commun Technol GCCT 2015*, 2015, 169–173, https://doi.org/10.1109/GCCT.2015.7342646.
5. Kelly, F.J., Fussell, J.C. "Improving IAQ, health and performance within environments where people live, travel, learn and work," *Atmos Environ*, 200, 2019, 90–109, https://doi.org/10.1016/j.atmosenv.2018.11.058.
6. Azam, A.G., Zanjani, B.R., Mood, M.B. "Effects of air pollution on human health and practical measures for prevention in Iran," 2016, https://doi.org/10.4103/1735-1995.189646.
7. Tham, K.W. "IAQ and its effects on humans – A review of challenges and developments in the last 30 years," *Energy Build*, 130, 2016, 637–650, https://doi.org/10.1016/j.enbu ild.2016.08.071.
8. NIOSH. *Nomination of welding fumes.* 2002. National Institute for Occupational Safety and Health.
9. Qolik, A. "Bahaya Asap dan Radiasi Sinar Las Terhadap Pekerja Las di Sektor Informal," *Jurnal Teknik Mesin Dan Pembelajaran* , 1, 2018, 1–4.
10. Popovi, O., Proki, R., Burzi, M., Belji, B. "Fume and gas emission during arc welding: Hazards and recommendation, Renewable and Sustainable Energy Reviews" *Renewable and Sustainable Energy Reviews*, 37, 2014, 509–516, https://doi.org/10.1016/j.rser.2014.05.076.

11. Serbula, S.M., Milosavljevic, J.S., Radojevic, A.A., Kalinovic, J.V., Kalinovic, T.S. "Science of the Total Environment Extreme air pollution with contaminants originating from the mining – metallurgical processes," *Sci Total Environ*, 2017, https://doi.org/10.1016/j.scitotenv.2017.02.091.

12. Pham V.T., Nguyen, T.P.N. "IAQ and health risk assessment for workers in packaging production factory, Can Tho city, Viet Nam", *Journal of Vietnamese Environment* 10, 2018, 66–71, https://doi.org/10.13141/jve.vol10.no2.pp66-71.

13. Al-zboon, K.K. "Indoor air quality in steel making industries," *Environmental Management and Sustainable Development*, 8, 2019,147–159, https://doi.org/10.5296/emsd.v8i1.14315.

14. Müller, D., Klingelhöfer, D., Uibel, S., Groneberg, D.A. "Car indoor air pollution – analysis of potential sources", *Journal of Occupational Medicine and Toxicology*, 2011, 1–7.

15. Cepeda, M., Schoufour, J., Freak-poli, R. "Levels of ambient air pollution according to mode of transport: a systematic review", *Lancet Public Health* 2016, 2667, https://doi.org/10.1016/S2468-2667(16)30021-4.

16. Karanasiou, A., Viana, M., Querol, X., Moreno, T., Leeuw, F. De. "Science of the Total Environment Assessment of personal exposure to particulate air pollution during commuting in European cities – Recommendations and policy implications," *Sci Total Environ*, 490, 2014, 785–797, https://doi.org/10.1016/j.scitotenv.2014.05.036.

17. Vanker, A., Barnett, W., Nduru, P.M., Gie, R.P., Sly, P.D., Zar, H.J. "Home environment and indoor air pollution exposure in an African birth cohort study," *Sci Total Environ*, 536, 2015, 362–367, https://doi.org/10.1016/j.scitotenv.2015.06.136.

18. Buthelezi, S.A., Kapwata, T., Wernecke, B., Webster, C., Mathee, A., Wright, C.Y. "Household fuel use for heating and cooking and respiratory health in a low-income, South African coastal community," *Int J Environ Res Public Health*, 16, 2019, https://doi.org/10.3390/ijerph16040550.

19. Chafe, Z.A., Brauer, M., Klimont, Z., Van Dingenen, R., Mehta, S., Rao, S., et al. "Household cooking with solid fuels contributes to ambient PM$_{2.5}$air pollution and the burden of disease," *Environ Health Perspect*, 122, 2015, 1314–1320, https://doi.org/10.1289/ehp.1206340.

20. Kampa, M., Castanas, E. "Human health effect of air polution-Environment Polution," *Environ Pollut*, 151, 2007, 362–367, https://doi.org/10.1016/j.envpol.2007.06.012.

21. Saad, S.M., Shakaff, A.Y.M., Saad, A.R.M., Yusof, A.M., Andrew, A.M., Zakaria, A., et al. "Development of indoor environmental index: Air quality index and thermal comfort index," *AIP Conf Proc*, 1808, 2017, https://doi.org/10.1063/1.4975276.

22. USEPA. *Data Quality Report* 2015.

23. Ogunbayo, A.O. *Retrospective study of effects of air pollution on human health*, 2016.

24. Brown, J.S., Gordon, T., Price, O., Asgharian, B. *Thoracic and respirable particle definitions for human health risk assessment*, 2013, 1–12.

25. Kim, K., Kabir, E., Kabir, S. "A review on the human health impact of airborne particulate matter," *Environ Int*, 74, 2015,136–143, https://doi.org/10.1016/j.envint.2014.10.005.

26. Mabahwi, N.A.B., Leh, O.L.H., Omar, D. "Human health and wellbeing: Human health effect of air pollution," *Procedia – Soc Behav Sci*, 153, 2014, 221–229, https://doi.org/10.1016/j.sbspro.2014.10.056.

27. Anwar, F., Chaudhry, F.N., Nazeer, S., Zaman, N., Azam, S. "Causes of ozone layer depletion and its effects on human: Review", *Atmospheric and Climate Sciences*, 2016, 129–134.

28. Mohanty, B. *Air pollution*, 2014.
29. Levy, R.J. "Neurotoxicology and teratology carbon monoxide pollution and neurodevelopment: A public health concern," *Neurotoxicol Teratol*, 49, 2015, 31–40, https://doi.org/10.1016/j.ntt.2015.03.001.
30. Programme EJR. *Environmental health criteria 213 carbon monoxide*, 2004.
31. Chen, T., Gokhale, J., Shofer, S., Kuschner, W.G. "Outdoor air pollution: Nitrogen dioxide, sulfur dioxide, and carbon monoxide health effects," *Med Sci*, 333, 2007, 249–256, https://doi.org/10.1097/MAJ.0b013e31803b900f.
32. Sharma, S.B., Jain, S., Khirwadkar, P., Kulkarni, S. "The effect of air pollution on the envirotment and human health," *Al Indian J Res Pharm Biotechnol*, 1, 2013, 2320–3471.
33. Panagopoulos, I.K., Karayannis, A.N., Kassomenos, P., Aravossis, K. "A CFD simulation study of VOC and formaldehyde indoor air pollution dispersion in an apartment as part of an indoor pollution management plan," 2011, 758–762, https://doi.org/10.4209/aaqr.2010.11.0092.
34. Fernández, L.C., Alvarez, F., González-barcala, F.J., Antonio, J., Portal, R. "Indoor air contaminants and their impact on respiratory pathologies", *Arch Bronconeumol*, 49, 2013, 22–27.
35. Tasdibi, D., Cevizci, S., Cotuker, O. "Association between respiratory health and indoor air pollution exposure in Canakkale, Turkey," *Build Environ*, 2015, https://doi.org/10.1016/j.buildenv.2015.01.023.
36. Shuai, J., Kim, S., Ryu, H., Park, J., Lee, C.K., Kim, G. "Health risk assessment of volatile organic compounds exposure near Daegu dyeing industrial complex in South Korea," 2018, 1–13.
37. Úlfrún V, Hellsing L. *IAQ in junior high schools in Reykjavik*, 2009.
38. Cui W, Cao G, Park JH, Ouyang Q, Zhu Y. "Influence of indoor air temperature on human thermal comfort, motivation and performance," *Build Environ*, 68, 2013, 114–122, https://doi.org/10.1016/j.buildenv.2013.06.012.
39. Xiong, J., Lian, Z., Zhou, X., You, J., Lin, Y. "Effects of temperature steps on human health and thermal comfort," *Build Environ*, 94, 2015, 144–154, https://doi.org/10.1016/j.buildenv.2015.07.032.
40. Davis, R.E., McGregor, G.R., Enfield, K.B. "Humidity: A review and primer on atmospheric moisture and human health," *Environ Res*, 144, 2016, 106–116, https://doi.org/10.1016/j.envres.2015.10.014.
41. Pflüger, R., Feist, W., Tietjen, A., Neher, A. "Physiological impairments at low indoor air humidity," *Gefahrstoffe Reinhaltung Der Luft*, 73, 2013, 107–108.
42. Schwartz, J., Samet, J.M., Patz, J.A. "Hospital admissions for heart disease: The effects of temperature and humidity," *Epidemiology*, 15, 2004, 755–761, https://doi.org/10.1097/01.ede.0000134875.15919.0f.
43. Nielsen, K.F., Holm, G., Uttrup, L.P., Nielsen, P.A. "Mould growth on building materials under low water activities. Influence of humidity and temperature on fungal growth and secondary metabolism," *Int Biodeterior Biodegrad*, 54, 2004, 325–336, https://doi.org/10.1016/j.ibiod.2004.05.002.
44. Kumar, N.S., Vuayalakshmi, B., Prarthana, R.J., Shankar, A. "IOT based smart garbage alert system using Arduino UNO," *IEEE Reg 10 Annu Int Conf Proceedings/TENCON*, 2017, 1028–1034, https://doi.org/10.1109/TENCON.2016.7848162.
45. Jacobs, D.E., Kelly, T., Sobolewski, J. "Linking public health, housing, and indoor environmental policy: Successes and challenges at local and federal agencies in the United States," *Environmental Health Perspectives*, 2007, 976–982, https://doi.org/10.1289/ehp.8990.

46. Khan, R., Khan, S.U., Zaheer, R., Khan, S. "Future internet: The Internet of things architecture, possible applications and key challenges," *Proc – 10th Int Conf Front Inf Technol FIT 2012*, 2012, 257–260, https://doi.org/10.1109/FIT.2012.53.

47. Idrees, Z., Zou, Z., Zheng, L. "Edge computing based IoT architecture for low cost air pollution monitoring systems: A comprehensive system analysis, design considerations & development," *Sensors (Switzerland)*, 2018, 18, https://doi.org/10.3390/s18093021.

48. Dhingra, S., Madda, R.B., Gandomi, A.H., Patan, R., Daneshmand, M. "Internet of things mobile-air pollution monitoring system (IoT-Mobair)," *IEEE Internet Things J*, 6, 2019, 5577–5584, https://doi.org/10.1109/JIOT.2019.2903821.

49. Chuyuan, Wei Y.L. "Design of energy consumption monitoring and energy-saving management system of intelligent building based on the Internet of things", *Int Con Elect Comm Control (ICECC)*, 2011, 3650–3652.

50. Jaladi, A.R., Khithani, K., Pawar, P., Malvi, K., Sahoo, G. "Environmental monitoring using wireless sensor networks (WSN) based on IOT," *Int Res J Eng Technol*, 4, 2017, 1371–1378.

51. Pasha, S. "Thingspeak based sensing and monitoring system for IoT with Matlab analysis," *Int J New Technol Res*, 2, 2016, 19–23, https://doi.org/ISSN: 2454–4116.

52. Borkar, C. *Development of wireless sensor network system for IAQ monitoring*, 2012.

53. Fan, X., Huang, H., Qi, S, Luo, X., Zeng, J., Xie, Q., et al. "Sensing home: A cost-effective design for smart home via heterogeneous wireless networks," *Sensors (Switzerland)*, 15, 2015, 30270–30292, https://doi.org/10.3390/s151229797.

54. Wang, Y., Chi, Z. "System of wireless temperature and humidity monitoring based on Arduino Uno platform," *Proc – 2016 6th Int Conf Instrum Meas Comput Commun Control IMCCC 2016*, 2016, 770–773, https://doi.org/10.1109/IMCCC.2016.89.

55. Samuel SSI. A review of connectivity challenges in IoT-smart home. 2016 3rd MEC Int Conf Big Data Smart City, *ICBDSC 2016*, 2016, 364–367, https://doi.org/10.1109/ICB DSC.2016.7460395.

56. Ott, W. *Air pollution indices: A compend*, 2014.

57. Kanchan, G.A.K., Goyal, P. "A review on air quality indexing system," *Asian J Atmos Environ*, 9, 2015, 101–113, https://doi.org/10.5572/ajae.2015.9.2.101.

58. Dionova, B.W., Mohammed, M.N., Al-Zubaidi, S., Yusuf, E. "Environment IAQ assessment using fuzzy inference system," *ICT Express*, 6, 2020, 185–194, https://doi.org/10.1016/j.icte.2020.05.007.

59. Mad Saad, S., Andrew, A.M., Shakaff, A.Y.M., Mohd Saad, A.R., Kamarudin, A.M.Y., Zakaria, A. "Classifying sources influencing IAQ (IAQ) using artificial neural network (ANN)," *Sensors (Switzerland)*, 15, 2015, 11665–11684, https://doi.org/10.3390/s15 0511665.

60. Lemeš, S. "Air Quality Index (AQI) – Comparative study and assessment of an appropriate model for B&H," *12th Sci Symp with Int Particip Metallic Nonmet Mater*, 2018, 282–291.

61. Viegas, C.V., Bond, A., Luis, J., Ribeiro, D., Maurício, P. "A review of environmental monitoring and auditing in the context of risk: unveiling the extent of a confused relationship," *J Clean Prod*, 2013, https://doi.org/10.1016/j.jclepro.2012.12.041.

62. Hapsari, A.A., Hajamydeen, A.I., Abdullah, M.I. "A Review on IAQ Monitoring using IoT at Campus Environment," *Int J Eng Technol*, 7, 2018, 55–60.

63. Kang, J., Hwang, K. "A Comprehensive real-time indoor air-quality level indicator", *Sustainability*, 2016, 1–15, https://doi.org/10.3390/su8090881.

64. Ben-David, T., Waring, M.S. "Impact of natural versus mechanical ventilation on simulated IAQ and energy consumption in offices in fourteen U.S. cities," *Build Environ*, 104, 2016, 320–336, https://doi.org/10.1016/j.buildenv.2016.05.007.

65. Stabile, L., Dell'Isola, M., Frattolillo, A., Massimo, A., Russi, A. "Effect of natural ventilation and manual airing on IAQ in naturally ventilated Italian classrooms," *Build Environ*, 98, 2016, 180–189, https://doi.org/10.1016/j.buildenv.2016.01.009.

66. Agency USE. "Peer review and supporting literature review of air sensor technology performance targets peer review and supporting literature," *Review of Air Sensor Technology Performance Targets*, 2018.

67. Kim, J.Y., Chu, C.H., Shin, S.M. "ISSAQ: An integrated sensing systems for real-time IAQ monitoring," *IEEE Sens J*, 14, 2014, 4230–4244, https://doi.org/10.1109/JSEN.2014.2359832.

68. Hapsari, A.A., Hajamydeen, A.I., Vresdian, D.J., Manfaluthy, M., Prameswono, L., Yusuf, E. "Real time Wireless Sensor Network (WSN) based IAQ monitoring system," *ICETAS*, 52, 2019, 324–327, https://doi.org/10.1016/j.ifacol.2019.12.430.

69. Zhi, S. "Intelligent controlling of IAQ based on remote monitoring platform by considering building environment," 2017, 627–31.

70. Lai, X., Yang, T., Wang, Z., Chen, P. "IoT implementation of Kalman Filter to improve accuracy of air quality monitoring and prediction," *Appl Sci*, 9, 2019, https://doi.org/10.3390/app9091831.

71. Esquiagola, J., Manini, M., Aikawa, A., Yoshioka, L., Zuffo, M. "SPIRI: Low power IoT solution for monitoring indoor air quality", The 3rd International Conference on Internet of Things, Big Data and Security – IoTBDS, 2018, 285–90.

72. He, J., Xu, L., Wang, P., Wang, Q. "A high precise E-nose for daily IAQ monitoring in living environment," *Integr VLSI J*, 58, 2017, 286–294, https://doi.org/10.1016/j.vlsi.2016.12.010.

73. Kumar, S. "Air quality monitoring system based on IoT using Raspberry Pi", *2017 Int Conf Comput Comm Aut (ICCCA)*, 2017, 1341–1346.

74. Gupta, H., Bhardwaj, D., Agrawal, H., Tikkiwal, V.A., Kumar, A. "An IoT based air pollution monitoring system for smart cities," *2019 IEEE Int Conf Sustain Energy Technol*, 2019, 173–177.

75. Firdhous, M.F.F., Sudantha, B.H., Karunaratne, P.M. "IoT Enabled Proactive IAQ Monitoring System for Sustainable Health Management", *2017 2nd Int Conf Comput Comms Tech (ICCCT)*, 2017, 216–221.

76. Asthana, P., Mishra, S. "IoT enabled real time bolt based IAQ monitoring system," *2018 Int Conf Comput Charact Tech Eng Sci*, 2019, 36–39, https://doi.org/10.1109/CCTES.2018.8674076.

77. Shah, H.N., Khan, Z., Merchant, A.A., Moghal, M., Shaikh, A., Rane, P. "IOT based air pollution monitoring system", *International Journal of Scientific & Engineering Research*, 9, 2018, 5–9.

78. Tapashetti, A., Vegiraju, D., Ogunfunmi, T. "IoT-enabled air quality monitoring device," *IEEE 2016 Glob Humanit Technol Conf*, 2016, 0–3.

79. Sabiq, A., Alfarisi, T. "Sistem Wireless Sensor Network Berbasis Arduino Uno dan Raspberry Pi untuk Pemantauan Kualitas Udara di Cempaka Putih Timur," *Jakarta Pusat. Citee*, 2017, 301–305.

80. Molka-Danielsen, J., Engelseth, P., Wang, H. "Large scale integration of wireless sensor network technologies for air quality monitoring at a logistics shipping base," *J Ind Inf Integr*, 10, 2018, 20–28, https://doi.org/10.1016/j.jii.2018.02.001.

81. Shah, J., Mishra, B. "Customized IoT enabled wireless sensing and monitoring platform for smart buildings," *Procedia Technol*, 23, 2016, 256–263, https://doi.org/10.1016/j.protcy.2016.03.025.

82. Mishra, A. "Air pollution monitoring system based on IoT: Forecasting and predictive modeling using machine learning," *Int Conf Appl Electromagn Signal Process Commun*, 2018.

83. Faroqi, A., Hadisantoso, E.P., Halim, D.K., Ws, M.S., Sains, F. "Perancangan Alat Pendeteksi Kadar Polusi Udara Mengunakan Sensor Gas Mq-7 Dengan Teknologi Wireless Hc-05," *Latar Belakang*, X, 2016, 33–47.

84. Bhattacharya, S., Sridevi, S.P.R. "IAQ monitoring using wireless sensor network," *Int Conf Sens Technol Indoor*, 172, 2012, 422–427, https://doi.org/10.21608/jsrs.2015.19949.

85. Tian, F.C., Kadri, C., Zhang, L., Feng, J.W., Juan, L.H., Na, P.L. "A novel cost-effective portable electronic nose for indoor/in-car air quality monitoring," *2012 Int Conf Comput Distrib Control Intell Enviromental Monit A*, 2012, https://doi.org/10.1109/CDCIEM.2012.9.

86. Alix, K.K.M., Lazatin, C.R.P., Waquiz, R.A.T. *Carbon monoxide monitoring and alert system for automobiles by 2013*.

87. Sun, W., Duan, N., Ji, P., Yao, R., Ma, C., Huang, J., et al. "Intelligent in-vehicle air quality management: A smart mobility application dealing with air pollution in the traffic", 23rd World Congress on Intelligent Transportation Systems Melbourne Australia, 2016, 10–4.

88. Kalantar-zadeh, K. *Investigation of gas sensors for 2017*.

89. Blaschke, M., Tille, T., Robertson, P., Mair, S., Weimar, U., Ulmer, H., et al. "MEMS gas-sensor array for monitoring the perceived car-cabin air quality," 6, 2006, 1298–1308.

90. Patil, S.S., Singh, P.J. "Monitoring and controlling of hazardous gases inside vehicle and alerting using gsm technology for the safety of people inside the vehicle", *International Journal of Science, Engineering and Technology*, 3, 2015, 238–243.

91. Devarakonda, S., Sevusu, P., Liu, H., Liu, R., Iftode, L., Nath, B. *Real-time air quality monitoring through mobile sensing in metropolitan areas*, 2013.

92. Alrazni, W.H.D. *Improving IAQ (IAQ) in Kuwaiti housing developments at design, construction, and occupancy stages*, 2016.

93. Hassan, A.S.M.R. "Natural ventilation of indoor air temperature: A case study of the traditional Malay house in Penang School of Housing, Building and Planning," *Sci Appl Publ Sci*, 3, 2010, 521–528.

94. Wang, Y., Luo, G., Geng, F., Li, Y., Li, Y. "Numerical study on dust movement and dust distribution for hybrid ventilation system in a laneway of coal mine," *J Loss Prev Process Ind*, 36, 2015, 146–157, https://doi.org/10.1016/j.jlp.2015.06.003.

95. Li, Y., He, J. *Design of an intelligent IAQ monitoring and purification device*, 2017, 1147–50.

96. Pradityo, F., Surantha, N. "IAQ monitoring and controlling system based on IoT and Fuzzy logic," 2019 *7th Int Conf Inf Commun Technol*, 2019, 1–6.

97. Aslam, Z., Khalid, W., Ahmed, T., Marghoob, D., *Microcontroller APIC. Automated control system for IAQ management*, 2017, 0–3.

98. Mohammed, M.N. "Investigation on Carbon Monoxide Monitoring and Alert System for Vehicles," *2019 IEEE 15th Int Colloq Signal Process Its Appl*, 2019, 239–242.

99. Yunus, S., Saini, M., Sultan, A.R., Nur, R., Program, D., Teknik, S., et al. *Pengaruh Ejektor Hasil Rancang Bangun Terhadap Pengurangan Gas 2018*, 2018, 47–52.

100. Nindi Meliyanto, B.E. "Pengendali Kipas Sirkulasi Udara Melalui Deteksi Suhu Udara Dan Kadar Karbondioksida Berlebih", *Jurnal Ilmiah Go Infotech*, 20, 2014, 1–8.

101. Widodo, S., Amin, M.M., Sutrisman, A., Putra, A.A. "Rancang Bangun Alat Monitoring Kadar Udara Bersih Dan Gas Berbahaya Co, Co2," *DAN CH4 DI DALAM*, 2017, 105–119.
102. Melo, W.N., Sompie, S., Allo, E.K. "Rancang Bangun Alat Pembersih Udara Dalam Ruang Tertutup Dengan Metode Ionisasi," 4, 2015, 67–77.
103. Schulze, T., Eicker, U. "Controlled natural ventilation for energy efficient buildings," *Energy Build*, 56, 2013, 221–232, https://doi.org/10.1016/j.enbuild.2012.07.044.
104. Dimitroulopoulou, C. "Ventilation in European dwellings: A review," *Build Environ*, 47, 2012, 109–125, https://doi.org/10.1016/j.buildenv.2011.07.016.
105. Pitarma, R. "Monitoring indoor air quality for enhanced occupational health", *Journal of Medical Systems*, 2017, https://doi.org/10.1007/s10916-016-0667-2.

5 Predictive Model for Brain Tumour Detection Based on IoT MRI Scan

Asmita Dixit and Aparajita Nanda
Jaypee Institute of Information Technology

CONTENTS

DOI: 10.1201/9781003146087-7

The formation of abnormal cells in the brain leads to the start of a brain tumour. If a tumour is large, but the growth rate is low, then that tumour is not that dangerous compared to the smaller tumour size but growing at a fast rate. Hence the detection of a brain tumour in the initial stages is essential. The tumour is generally divided into two types: cancerous (malignant) and benign. Though there are many methods available for brain tumour segmentation, most of them involve traditional hand-picking methods. This chapter presents fully automated methods which combine fuzzy c means and 3d active contour for tumour region segmentation. Fuzzy c means acts as a soft clustering technique, and snake's method has been used to identify the contour. Internet of things (IoT) is used for predicting whether a person needs surgeries depending upon the MRI.

5.1 INTRODUCTION

Brain tumour starts when normal cells acquire errors (mutations) in their Deoxyribonucleic Acid (DNA). These types of mutations allow cells to partition and grow at an increasingly exponential rate and continue to live when healthy cells eventually die. This results in a massive growth of mutated cells, which forms a tumour. People generally exposed to ionizing radiation have a high chance of being identified with a brain tumour. Different types of brain tumours exist; some are cancerous (malignant), while some are non-cancerous (benign). The growth rate and the location of the tumour define how it will affect our nervous system. e.g. a large tumour but is not growing is less dangerous than a small tumour in size and growing rapidly.

5.1.1 MRI vs CT Scan

Though CT scan is a fast technique and can provide images of organs and tissues and skeleton structure faster, MRIs are highly adept at capturing images.

MRI images make use of the magnetic field, whereas CT scan uses X-ray technology.

5.1.2 Diffused Low-Grade Gliomas

DLGGs are diffusely infiltrative essential cerebrum tumours. They speak to around 15% of essential cerebrum tumours and influence more youthful patients (somewhat a larger number of guys compared to females) than the most widely recognized glioblastomas (mean age around 38 years of age). They are characterized into three histological subtypes indicated by their prevalent c type of cell: oligodendrogliomas, oligoastrocytomas, and astrocytomas. A typical morphotype on histological investigation characterizes diffuse poor quality glioma. Nonetheless, these tumours display a wide heterogeneity in their level of natural aggressivity, bringing about an enormous scope of survival times. A few elements at the conclusion have been found to distinguish various subgroups of anticipation. Yet, there is developing proof that the natural elements of the tumour that can be assessed over a short introductory development assumes a noteworthy job in foreseeing the general forecast at an individual scale.

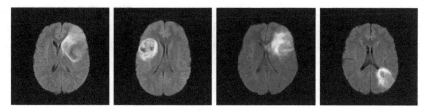

FIGURE 5.1   FLAIR T2 MR images of different DLGG.

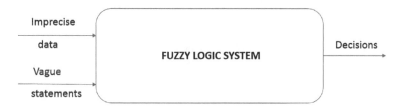

FIGURE 5.2   A fuzzy system that takes input as imprecise and vague data.

Figure 5.1 represents how flair T2 magnetic resonance images of different diffused low-gradeglioma look.

5.1.3   IoT PLATFORM

One of the famous cloud-based Internet of Things (IoT) platforms is thingspeak which was launched in 2010 and is used as a supporting service for IoT applications. This platform allows us to analyse, visualize and aggregate the live data stream on the cloud. It gives instant visualization for the data aggregated by the devices. It hence is used for proofing and prototyping all the concepts of the IoT system that generally demands analysis.

The platform is easy to configure for sending data just by using general IoT protocols. The visualization method collects the sensor data in real time. Then the data is collected from a third party in a process known as aggregation; after that, analysis is performed. After that a prototype is built without the server set up, automatic manipulation of data and communication by a third party is done.

5.1.4   FUZZY LOGIC

The Fuzzy Logic method, as shown in Figure 5.2, was first introduced in 1965, additionally by LotfiZadeh, and is a scientific instrument for managing vulnerability. It offers a delicate figuring organization that leads to a significant idea of figuring out patterns with words.

It furnishes a strategy to manage imprecision and data granularity. The fluffy hypothesis gives a component for speaking to semantic develops, for example, "some", "low"," medium", "frequently," and "maybe a couple" as a rule, and the fluffy rationale gives a deduction structure that empowers proper human thinking capacities. Despite what might be expected, the conventional two-fold set hypothesis portrays fresh occasions, occasions that either do or do not happen. The fuzzy value lies between 0 and 1, excluding 0 and 1, as it will lead to a crisp set. The value between 0 and 1 indicates the range of fuzziness that can be allowed.

5.1.5 ACTIVE CONTOUR

Dynamic shape or active contour can generally be characterized into parametric and geometric dynamic forms. The parametric dynamic forms are expressly spoken to as parameterized bends in the Lagrange formulation. They are delicate to the underlying shape and cannot normally deal with topological changes. At the same time, the geo-metric dynamic shapes are spoken to verifiable and develop as per the Euler plan dependent on the hypothesis of surface advancement and geometric streams.

The energy of contour is defined as submission of both internal and external energy, which is given by equation no. 1.

$$
\begin{aligned}
Energy_{snake}^{*} &= \int_0^1 Energy_{snake}\big(m(s)\big)ds \\
&= \int_0^1 \Big(E_{internal}\big(m(s)\big) + Energy_{image}\big(m(s)\big) + \big(m(s)\big)\Big)
\end{aligned}
\tag{1}
$$

Nonetheless, fuzzy c-means (FCM) implies anticipated tumour cells that are not anticipated by active contour (AC) calculation. The system gives a precise outcome when contrasted with active contour calculation. Even though unique fuzzy C-implies calculation yields great outcomes for sectioning commotion free pictures, it neglects to fragment loud pictures. In this manner, we get benefits by incorporating these two calculations to diminish the number of cycles, which influences execution time and gives an exact outcome in tumour location.

5.2 LITERATURE REVIEW

Numerous systems have been suggested to distinguish the mind tumour as of late. The suggested strategies can be comprehensively ordered into two, savvy based and non- shrewd based. The most remarkable keen based frameworks are fake neural systems, fluffy c implies, k-implies bunching and a half and half strategies. The most remarkable non-smart techniques incorporate thresholding and area development. In any case, there is no unmistakable partition between the two, and the two frameworks depend on each other for getting the best outcome.

The authors have presented a hybrid algorithm using k-mean clustering and fuzzy c-mean, followed by level set segmentation stage and thresholding to provide accurate results to detect brain tumours [1]. The authors have suggested that k-means takes minimal time for computation and fuzzy c-means have a high accuracy rate.

This chapter introduces a mix of skull stripping strategies and changed fluffy c-implies to fragment the tumour area [5]. After the procured picture is denoized, it is deprived of extra tissues on the external limits. It is additionally handled through the fluffy c-implies calculation. The outcomes were demonstrated to be better contrasted with the standard fluffy c-implies when connected on an example of 100 MRIs.

The creators have assessed mind tissue compartments in 72 solid volunteers between 18 and 81 years with quantitative MRI [3]. They consumed that the intracranial part of the white issue was altogether lower in the age classes over 59 years. The CSF portion expanded fundamentally with age, steady with past reports. The intracranial level of dark issues diminished fairly with age. However, there was no noteworthy contrast between the most youthful subjects and the subjects over 59. A covariance modification for the volume of hyperintensities did not modify the previous outcomes. The intracranial level of white issue volume was firmly associated with the rate volume of CSF. The finding of an exceptionally critical reduction with age in white issue, without a considerable decline in dark issue, is steady with ongoing neuropathological reports in people and nonhuman primates. The authors have suggested a similar approach. They have combined the fuzzy c means algorithm with the snake algorithm and have compared results based on various parameters of peak noise to signal ratio and root mean square error. The efficiency of the algorithm has been improved significantly.

All the above methods alone are not sufficient to segment tumours successfully. Some authors have suggested a hybrid approach that could lead to better results [4], but combining or making a hybrid algorithm using Active contour and much fewer people have approached FCM. Some of them who have approached this hybrid method use the normal version of FCM; here, we have tried to give a probabilistic approach to FCM so that centre selection would have less chance to fall in the trap of local minima.

5.3 METHODOLOGY

The division of images into different smaller parts for further studies is termed image segmentation [2]. This study will study the brain tumour images obtained from BRATS 2015 dataset available freely on the internet. To calculate the accuracy of our algorithm, we will be using Jaccard's measurement and dice coefficient. As we know, brain tumour tissue is divided into three major areas: cerebrospinal fluid, white matter and grey matter. The experiment was conducted on images by dividing them into these separate portions. We have compared the results of previously available traditional methods with semi-automated and fully automated methods during our experiment. Our algorithm has shown significant satisfying accuracy over all the available hybrid methods.

5.3.1 Adopted Method

In Figure 5.3, we have presented the adopted methodology for the experiment conducted in this chapter. All the steps have been described briefly in the below subsections.

5.3.1.1 De-noising
X-ray footage is ordinarily impure by removing influences of mathematician and Poisson noise. Far and away, most of the de-noising calculations expect additional

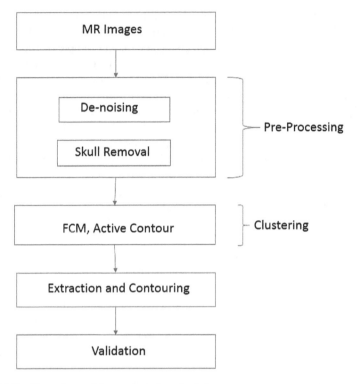

FIGURE 5.3   Flow chart of the suggested methodology.

substance mathematician clamour known as the racket. Few calculations are meant for mathematician clamour disposal, for instance, edge safeguarding reciprocal channel, complete selection, and non-neighbourhood implies. During this proposition, we tend to utilize the middle channel. Middle separating may be a nonlinear channel utilized as a viable technique for evacuating commotion whereas safeguarding edges. It works by moving element by pixel through the image, replacing every incentive with the centre advantage of neighbouring pixels. The instance of neighbours is understood because of the "window" that slides element by pixel over the full image. First, the middle is decided by first composing all the element esteems from the window into numerical request and replacing the element with the middle (median) pixel esteem. Image handling analysts typically attest that middle separation is superior to something direct separating for evacuating clamour at intervals at the sight of edges. The yield of this sub-venture in pre-process is the free noising MRI image.

5.3.1.2   Skull Removal

Picture foundation does not, for the most part, contain any helpful data but rather increment the preparing time [5]. Accordingly, expelling foundation, skull, eyes, skull, and all structures that are not in the intrigue decline the measure of the memory utilized and expanded the handling speed. Skull evacuated is finished by utilizing BSE (cerebrum surface extractor) calculation. The BSE calculation is utilized distinctly with MRI pictures. It channels the picture to expel abnormalities, identifies edges in the picture, and performs morphological disintegrations and mental detachment. It likewise performs surface clean-up and picture covering. The yield of this sub-step is the free noising MRI picture contains just the human cerebrum.

5.3.1.3 Fuzzy c Mean Algorithm

FCM is a grouping procedure that permits one snippet of data that has a place with at least two bunches. This system was found in 1974 by Dunn and upgraded in 1980 by Bezdek and is much of the time utilized in example acknowledgement. The primary part of this calculation works by allocating enrolment esteems to every datum guide subsequent toward each bunch focus based on separations between the group and the information point.

The higher the participation esteem the closer the information is to the bunch focus. The summation of participation of every datum point ought to be equivalent to 1. Figure 5.4 represents the flowchart of fuzzy c means algorithm that how the matrix is initialized, then we calculate or assume a random centre. We update u matric and based on certain equations the centre is updated. The steps of the algorithm are shown below.

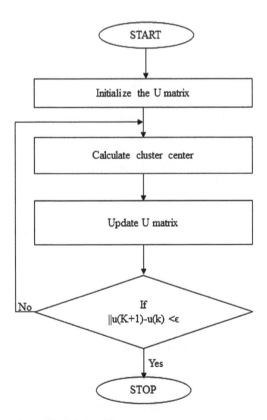

FIGURE 5.4 Flow chart of FCM algorithm.

Algorithm: FCM steps for centroid calculation

Step 1: Initialize A= $[A_{ij}]$ matrix, A^0

Step 2: At p-step: calculate the centre vectors $d^{(K)} = [d_j]$ with $A^{(K)}$ $d_j = \dfrac{\sum_{i=1}^{N} A_{ij}^m \cdot x_i}{\sum_{i=1}^{N} A_{ij}^m}$

Step 3: update A $^{(P)}$ and A $^{(P-1)}$ $A_{ij} = \dfrac{1}{\sum_{k=1}^{m} \left(\dfrac{\| x_i - m_j \|}{\| x_i - m_k \|} \right)^{\frac{2}{b-1}}}$

Step 4: If $\|A^{(P+1)} - A^{(P)}\| < \epsilon$

Step 5: Stop; or go to Step 2

Here, m is a real number $1 \le m \, \infty$

The algorithm will stop when $\max_{ij}$

$\|A^{(P+1)} - A^{(P)}\| < \epsilon$

Where ϵ will act as a conclusion criterion between 1 and 0, whereas p is the replication steps, this procedure leads to the convergence to a local minimum or a saddle point of J_m.

5.3.1.4 Probability-Based Segmentation

Besides the pre-processing step similitude assessing the group's list with their middle point, the accompanying advance is to stage the tumour from the MR picture by utilizing an exact edge [6]. The estimation of the edge impacts the assortment of the white added substances inside the two-fold picture. In the thresholding principally based division strategy, the MR picture is restored to dark in addition to the white picture. When the limit esteem is small scale, the range of the white added substances can be little, notwithstanding the tumour will never again be recognized or consequences. The tumour may be completely distinguished; however, it will show up a mess of white parts. So thought of characterizing proper likelihood esteem for additional exact recognition. $\delta = 0.6$, in which $\delta = 0.6$ the probability and "k" is previously defined. Suppose the hole among the pixel power esteem and the most astounding worth of the focuses is considerably less than δ. In that case, it is considered as a closer view or white pixel if now not, it is miles thought about as foundation or dark pixel.

5.4 THE ACTIVE CONTOUR MODEL (ACM)

The active contour system is specially designed for detecting blood vessels on coronary angiogram images for medical applications [7]. An active contour is essentially a curve made up of various energies. The curve deforms dynamically to mould to the shape of a targeted object. The energies in the active contour can be divided into two categories: external and internal. The function measuring the internal energy focuses mainly on the contour's intrinsic property, which leads to the measurement of elasticity and curvature of the contour. In contrast, the external energy functions are related to the image properties like contrast and brightness.

5.4.1 User Approximation

The algorithm that initiates contour with the user can construct approximately a rough contour that encloses the object that is to be tracked [10]. This contour is called the initial user approximation and hence can be of any shape and size. Instead of the user drawing the curve explicitly, the active contour algorithm makes the procedure simpler for the user by allowing him/her to click the points used to surround the object.

5.4.2 Internal Energy

The active contour's internal energy controls the curve shaping that eventually models the area of interest on a given image.

The properties of the internal energy can be further subdivided into two parts with individual weightings to influence the motion of the contour:

$$Einternal = \alpha.Eelastic + \beta.Ebending \qquad (2)$$

Where alpha and beta are constants and $E_{elastic}$ and $E_{bending}$ are given by below equations.

$$E_{elastic} = M_1 \sum_{i=1}^{Z} \left[\left(a_i - a_{i-1} \right)^2 + \left(b_i - b_{i-1} \right)^2 \right] \qquad (3)$$

$$E_{bending} = M_2 \sum_{i=1}^{Z} \left[\left(a_{i-1} - 2a_i - a_{i+1} \right)^2 + \left(b_{i-1} - 2b_i + b_{i+1} \right)^2 \right] \qquad (4)$$

The number of points used to form the contour is represented by Z, and i represent the index of the current point the calculation is focused on. M1 is a constant defined by the user, which affects similar to the constant corresponding to the strength of the spring. M2 is the user-defined constant, which affects similar to the constant corresponding to the spring's elasticity.

5.4.3 External Energy

The external energy of active contour depends on factors related to the image properties rather than the contour itself. Attributes such as noise level, brightness and contrast impose constraints that affect the motion but not the shape of the curve.

$$E_{image} = -k_3 * \Sigma \, image(x_i, \, y_i) \tag{5}$$

$$F_i x_i = \gamma * [image(x_{i+1}, \, y_i) - image(x_{i-1}, \, y_i)] \tag{6}$$

$$F_i y_i = \gamma * [image(x_i, \, y_{i+1}) - image(x_i, \, y_{i-1})] \tag{7}$$

where γ is related to the constant K3image (xi, yi) and defines the intensity value at the ith point of the contour.

5.4.4   THE TWO-PHASE FORMATION

$$E^{LIF}\left(\phi, h_1, h_2\right) = \lambda_1 \int \left[\int P_\sigma (r-y) \left| (y) - h_1(r) \right|^2 H\left(\phi(y)\right) dy \right] dr$$

$$\lambda_2 \int \left[\int P_\sigma (r-y) \left| I(y) - h_2(r) \right|^2 \left(1 - H\left(\phi(y)\right)\right) dy \right] dr \tag{8}$$

The above equation represents the two-phase active contour model [58].
   The Heavyside function is given by:

$$K_\epsilon\left(p\right) = \frac{1}{2}\left[1 + \frac{2}{\pi}arctan\left(\frac{p}{\epsilon}\right)\right] \tag{9}$$

The Dirac delta function is given by:

$$\delta_\epsilon\left(p\right) = H_\epsilon'\left(p\right) = \frac{1}{\pi}\frac{\epsilon}{\epsilon^2 + p^2} \tag{10}$$

5.5   RESULT

The GUI (graphical user interface) for the usage takes the client through generating the snake in a well-ordered fashion. In the initial step, the client chooses the picture and chooses the σ values responsible for the Gaussian smoothing. At that point, the client chooses the underlying snake's position by tapping on the picture and choosing control focuses that are later interjected (Spline based) into a contour. The client indicates different control parameters responsible for the formation of the snake.
   α(alpha): Determines the flexibility of the snake. It controls the strain in the form by joining with the main subsidiary term. β(beta): Indicates the inflexibility in the form by consolidating with the second subsidiary term. γ(gamma): step size is specified κ(kappa): Goes about as the scaling factor for the vitality term. W (Eline): Gauging factor for the power-based potential term. W (Edge): Gauging factor for the edge-based potential term. W (Eterm): Gauging factor for potential termination term.

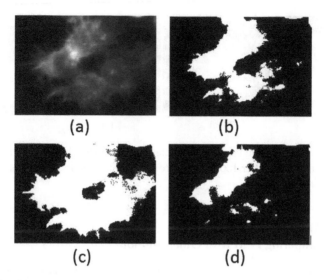

FIGURE 5.5 Segmentation using fuzzy c mean (a) is the original image (b) and (c) are intermediate steps (d) is the final image.

At that point, the client indicates the number of emphases for which the shape's position is to be computed. For the standard experiments given the task, predefined values for every one of the factors are hard-coded for comfort; however, they can be changed at any point.

Experiment 1:

α (alpha):0.50 β (beta):0.25 γ (gamma):1.00 κ(kappa): 0.25 W (Eline): 0.60, W (Edge):0.70, W (Eterm): 0.90

Experiment 1 demonstrates the use of the fuzzy c means algorithm. The above values have been set to reach the final result shown in Figure 5.5. This was a sample experiment performed in which the image was obtained from the internet. We have tested the image by applying the fuzzy c means algorithm twice on it, and at the end, a high pass filter has been used to enhance the properties of the image.

Experiment 2:

α(alpha):0.60 β (beta):0.15 γ (gamma):1.00 κ(kappa): 0.85 W (Eline): 0.30 W (Edge):0.20 W (Eterm): 0.9

AC algorithm on an image having tumour region. The AC algorithm can successfully mark the region having a tumour by using FCM to separate the tumour area, as shown in Figure 5.6.

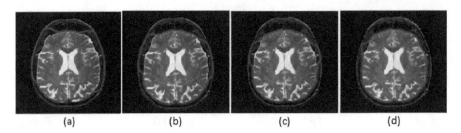

FIGURE 5.6 Segmentation using active contour (a) represents the image after 20 iterations (b) represents the image after 100 iterations (c) represents after 150 iterations (d) represents after 200 iterations.

TABLE 5.1
Comparing FCM with Other Methods

Method	Correlation	Structural Similarity
K-Mean(KM)	0.9526	1
Global Threshold	0.9456	1
Watershed	0.9823	1
Region Seed	0.9487	0.9586
Deformable Model	0.9452	0.9999
Morphological	0.91267	1

Table 5.1 represents the correlation and structural similarity between images when the tumour was segmented using various methods like the k-means clustering method, the global threshold method, watershed algorithm, the region seed growing algorithm, the deformable model and the morphological based model.

5.6 DISCUSSION

The fuzzy c means algorithm and the active contour algorithm [13] has performed well, and the mean squared error is also less and has shown significant improvement in PSNR.

On the off chance that the snake is introduced "excessively far" from the item limit, it is conceivable that the shape will most likely be unable to merge onto the object limit.

An expansion in smoothing expands the range from which a snake can meet onto an article smoothing. This can be viewed as that obscuring of edges increments their "encatchment" region. If the vitality scaling factor is "too huge" for a given picture, the dynamic form can meet the picture limit yet continues squirming along with the item limit. Much of the time, it winds up losing track of the article limit. W (Edge) esteem must be painstakingly picked if there should arise twofold pictures that have extremely high inclination esteems.

The Eterm characterizes the commitment of arches to the general vitality term. When weight related to this part is overwhelming in the general vitality, the snakes are by all accounts pulled into corners first before uniting onto the article limit. In situations where its weight is not overwhelming, edges are followed before the corners by the snake.

5.7 EVALUATION METRIC

Four metrics are used here to evaluate the results, i.e. dice coefficient (D), mean squared error (MSE), peak signal to noise ratio (PSNR), Tanimoto coefficient (T). The results of the experiment conducted have been presented in the form of tables below.

5.7.1 THE DICE COEFFICIENT

The Sørensen–Dice coefficient is a statistic used for comparing the similarity of two samples.

$$D = \frac{\left(2 * T_r P\right)}{\left(2 * T_r P + F_p P + F_p N\right)} \tag{11}$$

where, $F_p P = T_r P = TruePositiveFalsePositiveF_p N = FalseNegative$

As we can see from Table 5.2, the MSE when FCM algorithm is alone used to detect brain tumour compared with when we have combined active contour methodology with fuzzy technique.

The graph in Figure 5.7 represents an independent comparison between Active contour algorithm performance and FCM based on Dice index, false negative rate, which leads to under segmentation of tumour, false positive rate, leading to over-segmentation of tumour and the overlapped area.

5.7.2 TANIMOTO COEFFICIENT

The Tanamito coefficient between two distinct points p and q having m dimensions is calculated using the given equation no. 12.

TABLE 5.2
Performance Comparison Using MSE

Input Image	MSE	
	FCM	Active Contour and FCM
Brain.tif	0.1738	0.0554
Neuro.tif	0.1497	0.0441
Square.tif	0.1134	0.0845

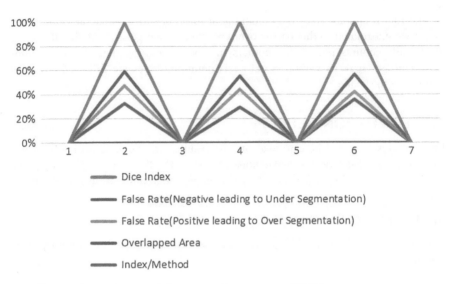

FIGURE 5.7   Comparison graph between active contour and FCM.

TABLE 5.3
Table Comparing FCM and Active Contour

Index /Method	Overlapped Area	False Rate (positive)	False Rate (Negative)	Dice Index
MatchingTemplate	0.549	0.245	0.195	0.685
Active(AC) contour	0.512	0.265	0.198	0.777
Automated Growth Region	0.647	0.123	0.257	0.785

$$T = \frac{\sum_{J=1}^{m} p_j q_j}{\sum_{j=1}^{m} p_j^2 + \sum_{j=1}^{m} q_j^2 - \sum_{j=1}^{m} p_j q_j} \tag{12}$$

The Tanimoto closeness is appropriate for a double factor, and parallel factors, the Tanimoto coefficient ranges from 0 to +1 (where +1 is the most elevated similitude).

Table 5.3 shows the comparison between FCM and active contour (AC). The final product of the improved probability-based division approach is in correlation with the mixes of improved probability-based fuzzy c-means and active shape di-vision strategies. In this assessment, the similarity of the ground truth picture and distinctive watched portioned pictures are assessed.

5.8 CONCLUSION

From the results and their discussion, we can see that the hybrid algorithm has performed very well. The performance has been evaluated on the basic of Dice coefficient, the peak signal to noise ratio parameter, and mean squared error parameter. We can see the comparison in the graphs and tables in the result section. Many algorithms perform well and give an accuracy of around 90–92 %, but with this hybrid approach, we have achieved an accuracy of around 94.3%. Hence, we can conclude that we can merge many algorithms to increase the efficiency and accuracy of segment brain tumours. The experiment for this chapter was conducted on a very limited number of images, but in future we plan to run the algorithm on the latest BRATS dataset or 3D MRI scans [9,11]. The future aspect of this chapter can lead to brain tumour classification using the recent CNN [8] and deep neural network approach [14].

REFERENCES

1. Abdel-Maksoud, Eman, Elmogy, Mohammed, Al-Awadi, Rashid. "Brain tumour segmentation based on a hybrid clustering technique," *Egyptian Informatics Journal* 16(1), 2015, 71–81.
2. Archip, Neculai, Jolesz, Ferenc A., Warfield, Simon K. "A validation framework for brain tumour segmentation," *Academic Radiology* 14(10), 2007, 1242–1251.
3. Atkins, M. Stella, and Mackiewich, Blair T. "Fully automatic segmentation of the brain in MRI," *IEEE Transactions on Medical Imaging* 17(1), 1998, 98–107.
4. You, Suhang, Tezcan, Kerem C., Chen, Xiaoran, Konukoglu, Ender. "Unsupervised lesion detection via image restoration with a normative prior," in *International Conference on Medical Imaging with Deep Learning*, 2019, pp. 540–556. PMLR.
5. Bilenia, Aniket, Sharma, Daksh, Raj, Himanshu, Raman, Rahul, Bhattacharya, Mahua. "Brain tumour segmentation with skull stripping and modified fuzzy C-means," in *Information and Communication Technology for Intelligent Systems*, 2019, pp. 229–237. Springer, Singapore.
6. Cahall, Daniel E., Rasool, Ghulam, Bouaynaya, Nidhal C., Fathallah-Shaykh, Hassan M. "Inception modules enhance brain tumour segmentation." *Frontiers in Computational Neuroscience* 13, 2019, 44.
7. Chan, Tony F., Vese, Luminita A.. "Active contour and segmentation models using geometric PDE's for medical imaging," in *Geometric Methods in Bio-medical Image Processing*, 2002, pp. 63–75. Springer, Berlin, Heidelberg.
8. Chang, Jie, Zhang, Luming, Gu, Naijie, Zhang, Xiaoci, Ye, Minquan, Yin, Rongzhang, Meng, Qianqian. "A mix-pooling CNN architecture with FCRF for brain tumour segmentation," *Journal of Visual Communication and Image Representation* 58, 2019, 316–322.
9. Cheng, Heng-Da, Jiang, X.H., Sun, Ying, Wang, Jingli. "Color image segmentation: advances and prospects," *Pattern Recognition* 34(12), 2001, 2259–2281.
10. Clark, Matthew C., Hall, Lawrence O., Goldgof, Dmitry B., Velthuizen, Robert, Murtagh, F. Reed, Silbiger, Martin S. "Automatic tumour segmentation using knowledge-based techniques," *IEEE Transactions on Medical Imaging* 17(2), 1998, 187–201.
11. Cobzas, Dana, Birkbeck, Neil, Schmidt, Mark, Jagersand, Martin, Murtha, Albert. "3D variational brain tumour segmentation using a high dimensional feature set," in *2007 IEEE 11th International Conference on Computer Vision*, 2007, pp. 1–8. IEEE.

12. Corso, Jason J., Sharon, Eitan, Yuille, Alan. "Multilevel segmentation and integrated Bayesian model classification with an application to brain tumour segmentation," in *International Conference on Medical Image Computing and Computer-Assisted Intervention*, 2006, pp. 790–798. Springer, Berlin, Heidelberg.

13. Derraz, Foued, Beladgham, Mohamed, Khelif, M'hamed. "Application of active contour models in medical image segmentation," in *International Conference on Information Technology: Coding and Computing, 2004. Proceedings. ITCC 2004*, 2004, vol. 2, pp. 675–681. IEEE.

14. Dong, Hao, Yang, Guang, Liu, Fangde, Mo, Yuanhan, Guo, Yike. "Automatic brain tumour detection and segmentation using u-net based fully convolutional networks," in *Annual Conference on Medical Image Understanding and Analysis*, 2017, pp. 506–517. Springer, Cham.

6 A Comparative Analysis of Parametric and Non-Parametric Video Object Segmentation Methods for IoT and Other Applications Areas

Chandrajit M. and Vasudev T.
Maharaja Research Foundation
Maharaja Institute of Technology Mysore

Shobha Rani N. and Manohar N.
Department of Computer Science
Amrita School of Arts and Science, Mysuru Campus
Amrita

CONTENTS

Video object segmentation is the task of extracting the moving objects in video frames. This task is an essential task due to the varied number of real-time applications such as medical imaging in healthcare, automated surveillance, automated driver-assist system, behaviour analysis, gait recognition, drones, etc. The increased potential of

DOI: 10.1201/9781003146087-8

Internet of Things (IoT) to process video sequences effortlessly makes video object segmentation seemingly applicable for various IoT-based applications. In literature, we can find numerous works in this direction. However, the focus of this chapter is to comparatively analyse the techniques specific to parametric and non-parametric statistical hypothesis testing tools for video object segmentation. Two methods in each category are chosen for comparative analysis, and these methods are based on temporal differencing combined with statistical hypothesis testing tools. Further, we present a suitability study of the video object segmentation techniques for real-time applications.

6.1 INTRODUCTION

The rapid development in video technology has opened up huge requirements for a variety of computer vision-based applications. The majority of applications primarily rely on objects of interest for further analysis. The objects of interest in this scenario are the moving objects in video frames. Segmentation of moving objects is the initial task of any vision application. Generally, segmentation is achieved by background subtraction, optical flow, and temporal differencing based techniques. Due to the potential of deep networks, some of the works [16, 24, 28, 31] apply the deep network for video object segmentation. The background subtraction method consists of two steps. In the first step, a background image is generated by observing the pixel values of the initial frames of the video. Generally, the background image is constructed dynamically using a probability distribution. In the second step, an image subtraction operation is performed for foreground object segmentation. Flow vectors from successive frames of video are used to detect moving objects in the optical flow method. Successive frame subtraction is employed for moving object segmentation in the temporal differencing method. Gaussian Mixture Model for background construction and subsequent segmentation of moving objects using a threshold is discussed [29]. A combination of local pixel and block pixel features for background construction is explored in [7]. The ensemble of texture and edge features for pedestrian segmentation using background construction is discussed [3]. Kernel-based density estimation for background construction to segment moving objects is proposed in [13]. Moving object segmentation in the temporal domain with background subtraction is explored in [27]. Robust motion segmentation using Wronskian model-based background subtraction is discussed in [30]. A semi-supervised convolution network-based background subtraction is explored in [28]. Two-step based moving object segmentation comprising neural network and memory module to learn the object variations is proposed in [24]. A convolution neural network that learns the object appearance and motion for moving object segmentation is proposed [16]. A reinforcement-based model for video object segmentation is proposed in [31]. The authors in [12] proposed an optical flow-based method for motion segmentation. Two methods based on optical flow for moving object segmentation are reported in [32]. In the first method, expansion, shear and rotation are computed by the Jacobian matrix of the first spatial derivatives. In the second method, local properties of optical flow that are invariant to linear transformation are explored. Moving objects segmentation in mono and stereo cameras based on motion analysis of optical flow is proposed in [18]. The authors in [22] proposed a temporal differencing based method for motion segmentation. Temporal differencing with graph-cut based moving object segmentation is proposed in [20].

Further, the authors addressed the moving object segmentation in a non-stationary camera. A local adaptive temporal differencing based method for moving object segmentation is explored in [19]. Frame differencing combined with corner features for moving object segmentation in a meeting room is discussed in [2]. The authors in [10] proposed temporal based motion segmentation in the frequency transformed domain. The authors in [21] discussed an information theory-based temporal differencing motion segmentation method. The insights of the methods discussed for video object segmentation is presented in Table 6.1.

From Table 6.1, it can be noted that the solution to the problem of video object segmentation by satisfying the various constraints is highly challenging. Each method has its own set of pros and cons and thus clearly indicates the potential in this direction for further research due to the varied applications ranging from biometrics to the IoT-based drone.

Perhaps, achieving a promising solution for motion segmentation is quite challenging due to various factors such as noise in video capture, cluttered background, and dynamic environment, illumination variations, diverse sensors, etc., [1, 3, 4, 23, 26, 33].

Amongst the techniques for motion segmentation, temporal differencing is appropriate for a dynamic environment since it does not rely on background construction for segmentation. The methods are based on temporal differencing segment video objects by analysing the variation of pixel intensity values between two or three consecutive frames. Statistical hypothesis testing methods are employed in these techniques for ascertaining the variation.

TABLE 6.1
Comparative Analysis

Method	Can Handle Dynamic Environment	Can Handle Cluttered Environment	Accuracy of Segmentation	Computational Complexity	Sensor Suitability
Background Subtraction	✓	☐	High	Fair	Aerial, Night vision, Thermal
Optical Flow	☐	☐	High	High	Aerial, Night Vision, Thermal PTZ
Temporal Differencing	✓	✓	Low	Low	Aerial, Night Vision, Thermal PTZ
Deep Network	☐	✓	High	High	Aerial, Night Vision, Thermal PTZ

The field of statistics consists of tools for describing the data values, which we call descriptive statistics. On the other hand, statistics consist of tools to determine inferences about the data values we call inferential statistics. Statistical hypothesis testing is the most common method in inferential statistics. Hypothesis testing methods can be categorized as parametric and non-parametric [11, 15].

Parametric methods assume data values to be normal distribution and are based on fixed parameters for determining the probability model. T-Test, ANOVA, Z-Test, Hotelling's T-Square-Test, etc., are examples of parametric tests. Contrarily, non-parametric methods do not assume parameters or distribution for determining the probability model. The Kolmogorov–Smirnov test, Chi-Square test, Median test, etc., are examples of the non-parametric test [11, 17, 25]. This study will compare and contrast two methods, each in parametric and non-parametric domains proposed for video object segmentation. Under the parametric category, the T-Test based method proposed in [5] and modified Hotelling's T-Square test-based method proposed in [8] is chosen. Similarly, under the non-parametric category, the Chi-Square test-based method [7] and Kolmogorov–Smirnov test-based method [6] are chosen.

In this comparative analysis, we provide an overview of the methodology for segmentation in the next section. Then, we provide a detailed discussion on the experimental results of these four methods with evaluation metrics, and conclude with the summary.

6.2 OVERVIEW OF THE METHODOLOGY FOR MOTION SEGMENTATION

This section describes the generic methodology of video object segmentation methods that is reviewed in this work. Figure 6.1 presents the block diagram of the generic model. The methods use the statistical tests viz., T-Test, modified Hotelling's T-square test, Chi-Square test, and Kolmogorov–Smirnov (KS) test for video object segmentation inference on pixel values from consecutive frames.

Input frames are initially preprocessed to reduce the sensor noise using a Gaussian filter.

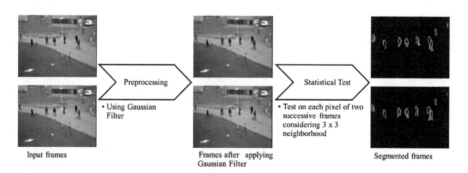

FIGURE 6.1 Generic methodology of temporal video object segmentation method.

$$G(x,y) = \frac{1}{2\pi\sigma^2} e^{-\frac{x^2+y^2}{2\sigma^2}} \tag{1}$$

where, x and y are the distances from the origin in the x and y-axis, and σ represents the standard deviation of the Gaussian distribution.

Subsequently, the mean of RGB is considered as colour space, and 3 x 3 pixel neighbourhood from successive frames is given as input to the statistical hypothesis test to determine variation among pixel values. A hypothesis test is a statistical test used to estimate the relationship between two populations described by variables. Also, it is used to estimate the likelihood of the hypothesis. In this context, the hypothesis test is used to observe the difference between neighbourhood pixel values of consecutive frames. A pixel is considered either a foreground pixel or a background pixel based on the measured difference value.

T-Test based video object segmentation is achieved using the following equation.

$$t_{P(w,h)} = \frac{\mu_{N9}^t - \mu_{N9}^{t+1}}{\sqrt{\dfrac{S_t^2 + S_{t+1}^2}{9}}} \tag{2}$$

Modified Hotelling's test-based video object segmentation is achieved by applying the following equation.

$$t^2 = \frac{n_1 n_2}{n_1 + n_2} \frac{\left(\mu_{N9}^t - \mu_{N9}^{t+1}\right)^2}{cov_{t,t+1}} \tag{3}$$

Chi-Square test-based video object segmentation is achieved by applying the following equation.

$$\chi_{P(w,h)}^2 = \sum_{k=1}^{9} \frac{\left(O_{P_{N9(RGB)_k}} - E_{P_{N9(RGB)_k}}\right)^2}{E_{P_{N9(RGB)_k}}} \tag{4}$$

where, $\chi_{P(w,h)}^2$ is the Chi-Square test statistic for each pixel.

KS test-based video object segmentation is achieved by applying the following equation.

$$D_{F_t, F_{t+1}} = \sup_x \left| F_{tP_{N9(RGB)}} - F_{t+1 P_{N9(RGB)}} \right| \tag{5}$$

where D is the KS test statistic for each pixel and sup is the supremum function.

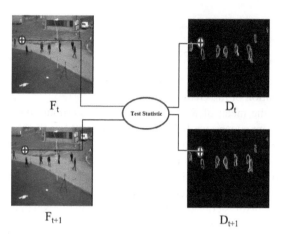

FIGURE 6.2   Test statistic computations.

Finally, the video objects are segmented based on test statistics with a predefined threshold, as shown in Figure 6.2. The reviewed methods do not apply any post-processing techniques for image enhancement.

The frames D_t and D_{t+1} are the resultant frames which contain foreground moving objects.

$$D_{P(w,h)_m} = \{RGB \, of \, F_{P(w,h)_m} \; (if \, T \geq \tau) \, 0 \qquad\qquad (otherwise) \qquad\qquad (6)$$

where, $m = \{t, t+1\}$ and $I_{P(w,h)}$ is the pixel in the input frame.

6.3   RESULTS AND DISCUSSION

The methods are tested on the benchmark PETS and Change Detection (CD) dataset. Figures 6.3–6.7 illustrates the qualitative results for the various dataset used for experimentation. The first row of the figure indicates the input frames, the second row of the figure indicates the results of the T-Test based method, the third row indicates the output of modified Hotelling's test-based method, the fourth row of the figure indicates the results of Chi-Square test-based method and fifth row of the figure indicates the results of KS test-based method. Experiments on thermal, PTZ, aerial, and night vision sensor videos have been conducted to test the efficacy of various sensor types. As per the qualitative analysis, we can infer that all the methods segment video objects satisfactorily in varied environments and sensors. Further, it is very difficult to compare the results with a human expert.

It can be noticed that there are some holes generated in the segmented objects in Figure 6.4 and Figure 6.6. This has resulted since the accuracy of segmentation by the temporal differencing based method is not that promising. Therefore, a post-processing technique may be applied to improve the results. This will help in accurate

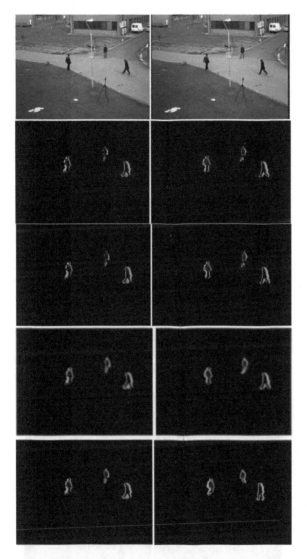

FIGURE 6.3   PETS 2013 People Tracking frames.

feature extraction for further analysis. The results for the night vision sensor presented in Figure 6.5 shows that the algorithm has failed to segment the object accurately, and the results are over segmented. This has happened due to the rapid movement of the vehicles and lights beamed on the road by the vehicles in the video. Working on this type of video is highly challenging, and hybrid techniques must be applied to accurately extract the objects. Contrary, the background subtraction based method will handle these situations efficiently as the camera is static. Therefore, the background can be modelled for object segmentation in these situations.

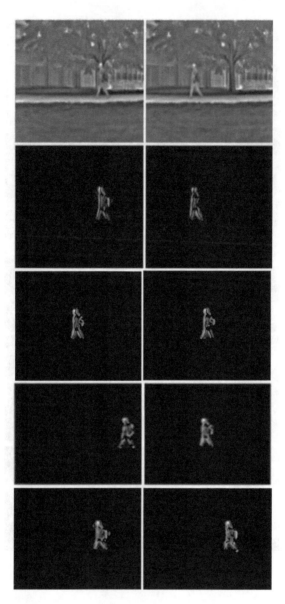

FIGURE 6.4   CD thermal frames.

Results of the quantitative analysis presented in Table 6.2 are measured using the precision, recall, and F-measure performance metrics. The graphical representation is given in Figure 6.8.

$$Precision = \frac{TP}{TP + FP} \tag{7}$$

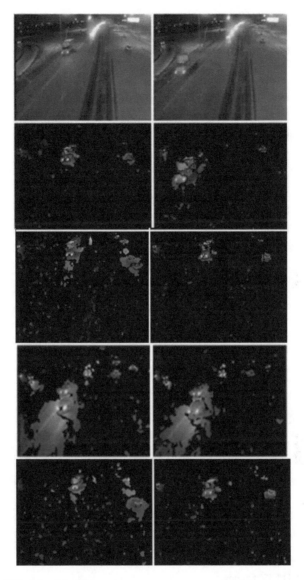

FIGURE 6.5 CD night vision frames.

$$Recall = \frac{TP}{TP + FN} \qquad (8)$$

$$F - measure = \frac{2 \times Precision \times Recall}{Precision + Recall} \qquad (9)$$

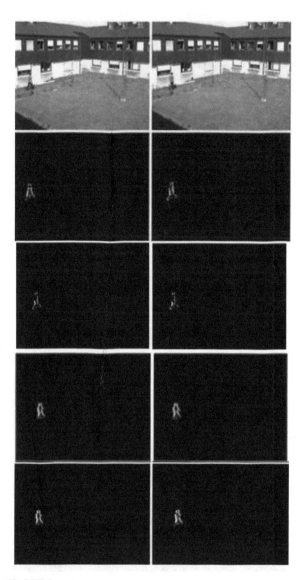

FIGURE 6.6   CD PTZ frames.

where *TP* is the pixels rightly categorized as foreground pixels, *FP* is the pixels falsely categorized as the foreground pixels, and *FN* is the measure of pixels belonging to the foreground but incorrectly categorized as background. The fraction of relevant instances are termed *precision*, whereas the fraction of relevant instances retrieved is called *recall*. The *F − measure* is the harmonic mean of *precision* and *recall* [14].

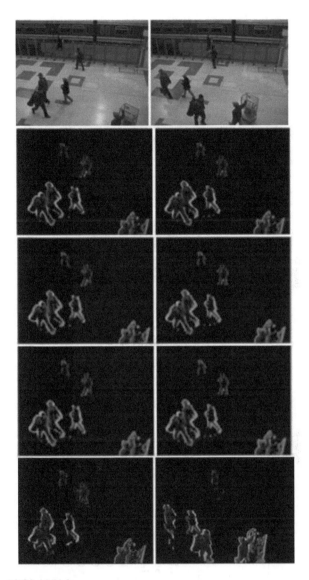

FIGURE 6.7 PETS 2006 frames.

From Table 6.2, it can be noted that all the methods reviewed are promising in near to accurate video object segmentation. Further, the non-parametric KS test and Chi-Square based methods perform significantly better compared to parametric counterparts. The highest and lowest F-measure of 0.78 and 0.58 respectively is achieved by KS test-based method. On the other hand, the lowest F-measure score is achieved by parametric methods.

TABLE 6.2
Quantitative Analysis

Dataset	Precision				Recall				F-measure			
	KS-Test	Chi-Square Test	T-Test	Modified Hotelling's T-Square Test	KS-Test	Chi-Square Test	T-Test	Modified Hotelling's T-Square Test	KS-Test	Chi-Square Test	T-Test	Modified Hotelling's T-Square Test
PETS 2013	0.79	0.76	0.66	0.73	0.75	0.71	0.62	0.68	0.77	0.73	0.64	0.70
PETS 2006	0.86	0.83	0.80	0.77	0.72	0.68	0.51	0.66	0.78	0.75	0.62	0.71
CD night vision sensor	0.54	0.51	0.47	0.47	0.63	0.60	0.49	0.53	0.58	0.55	0.47	0.50
CD PTZ	0.63	0.59	0.56	0.33	0.6	0.57	0.50	0.50	0.61	0.58	0.51	0.40
CD thermal sensor	0.81	0.78	0.66	0.77	0.69	0.65	0.59	0.61	0.75	0.71	0.62	0.67

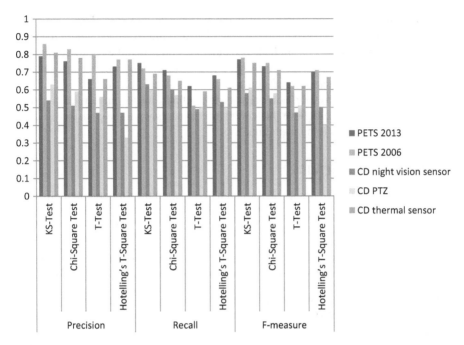

FIGURE 6.8 Graphical representation.

TABLE 6.3
Computation Time

Method	Average Time in ms
KS Test	145
Chi-Square	120
T-Test	50
Modified Hotelling's	50

Typically, this is due to the non-assumption nature of non-parametric methods concerning the distribution. Therefore, non-parametric based methods are suitable for video object segmentation for various sensors.

The approximate time required for video object segmentation for the methods is presented in Table 6.3. The size of the image used for computation is 340 x 260 pixels.

The test was carried out using C++ with OpenCV on the Intel Core i3 machine. It can be noted that there is a trade-off between computation time and accuracy.

6.4 CONCLUSION

In this chapter, a comparative analysis of statistical methods for video object segmentation is presented. The methods are based on statistical modelling combined with the temporal domain. The viability of using parametric and non-parametric statistical hypothesis testing tools both in the univariate and multivariate domain for video object segmentation has been studied. The outcomes infer that the reviewed methods satisfactorily segment the foreground objects in a relatively challenging environment.

Amongst the four methods, the non-parametric statistics based methods perform significantly better. Therefore, non-parametric methods are recommended for video object segmentation. We believe this comparative analysis will help further research in this direction by providing useful insights.

ACKNOWLEDGEMENT

The authors acknowledge Maharaja Research Foundation for support and motivation.

REFERENCES

1. Ahn J., Choi C., Kwak S., Kim K., Byun H. "Human tracking and silhouette extraction for human robot interaction systems," *Pattern Analysis and Applications*, 12(2), 2009, 167–177.
2. Algethami, N., Redfern, S. "Combining accumulated frame differencing and corner detection for motion detection," *EG UK Computer Graphics & Visual Computing*, 2018, 7–14, DOI: 10.2312/cgvc.20181202.
3. Armanfard, N., Komeili, M., Kabir, E. "Ted: A texture-edge descriptor for pedestrian detection in video sequences," *Pattern Recognition*, 45(3), 2012, 983–992.
4. Armanfard, N., Komeili, M., Valizade, M., Kabir, E., Jalili, S. "A non-parametric pixel-based background modeling for dynamic scenes", in 2009 International Conference on Advances in Computational Tools for Engineering Applications, 2009, pp. 369–373. IEEE.
5. Chandrajit, M., Girisha, R., Vasudev, T. "Motion segmentation from surveillance videos using T-test statistics," in *Proceedings of the 7th ACM India Computing Conference (COMPUTE '14)*, 2014. ACM. Article 2, 10 pages. DOI=http://dx.doi.org/10.1145/2675744.2675748.
6. Chandrajit, M., Vasudev, T., Shobha Rani, N. "Moving object segmentation from surveillance video sequences: A non-parametric approach," in *Proceedings of the International Conference on Signal and Image Processing*, 2017 (ICSIP '17).
7. Chandrajit, M., Girisha, R., Vasudev, T. "Motion segmentation using Chi-square test statistics," in *Proceedings of the 2nd International Conference on – (ERCICA 2014)*, vol. 2, 2014, pp. 365–372. Elsevier.
8. Chandrajit, M., Girisha, R., Vasudev, T. "Motion segmentation using modified Hotelling's T-square test statistics," *IJIGSP*, 8(7), 2016, 41–48, DOI: 10.5815/ijigsp.2016.07.05.
9. Chen, Y., Chen, C., Huang, C., Hung. Y. "Efficient hierarchical method for background subtraction," *Pattern Recognition*, 40(10), 2007, 2706–2715.
10. Cheng, F., Chen, Y., "Real time multiple objects tracking and identification based on discrete wavelet transform," *Pattern Recognition*, 39(6), 2006, 1126–1139.
11. David, A.R. *Statistics for Business and Economics*, 11th edn, 2012. Cengage Learning.
12. Denman, S., Fookes, C., Sridharan S. "Improved simultaneous computation of motion detection and optical flow for object tracking," in *Proceedings of the International Conference on Digital Image Computing: Techniques and Applications*, 2009, pp. 175–182. DICTA.

13. Elgammal, A., Duraiswami, R., Harwood, D., Davis L. "Background and foreground modeling using non-parametric kernel density estimation for visual surveillance," *Proceedings of the IEEE*, 90(7), 2002, 1151–1163.

14. Goyette, N., Jodoin, P., Porikli, F., Konrad, J., Ishwar P. "Changedetection.net: A new change detection benchmark dataset," in *Proceedings of the IEEE Computer Society Conference on Computer Vision and Pattern Recognition Workshops*, 2012, pp. 1–8. IEEE.

15. Gupta, S.C. *Fundamentals of Statistics*, 2009. Himalaya Publishing House.

16. Jeong, J., Yoon, T.S., Park, J.B. "MOSnet: moving object segmentation with convolutional networks," *Electronics Letters, IET Digital Library*, 54(3), 2018, 136–138.

17. Johnson R.A., Winchern D.W. *Applied Multivariate Statistical Analysis*, 2007. Pearson Prentice Hall.

18. Klappstein, J., Vaudrey, T., Rabe, C., Wedel, A., Klette R. "Moving object segmentation using optical flow and depth information," in Wada T., Huang F., Lin S. (eds.), *Advances in Image and Video Technology. PSIVT 2009. Lecture Notes in Computer Science*, vol. 5414, 2009, pp. 611–623. Springer. https://doi.org/10.1007/978-3-540-92957-4_53.

19. Le, X., Gonzalez, R. "Hybrid salient motion detection using temporal differencing and Kalman filter tracking with non-stationary camera," *Proceedings of the IEEE International Conference on Image Processing (ICIP)*, 2017, pp. 3345–3349. IEEE. doi: 10.1109/ICIP.2017.8296902.

20. Lim, T., Han, B., Han, J.H. "Modeling and segmentation of floating foreground and background in videos," *Pattern Recognition*, 45(4), 2012, 1696–1706.

21. Liu, C., Yuen, P.C., Qiu. G. "Object motion detection using information theoretic spatio temporal saliency," *Pattern Recognition*, 42(11), 2009, 2897–2906.

22. Murali, S., Girisha, R. "Segmentation of motion objects from surveillance video sequences using temporal differencing combined with multiple correlation", in *Proceedings of the Sixth IEEE International Conference on Advanced Video and Signal Based Surveillance (AVSS)*, 2009, pp. 472–477. IEEE.

23. Olatunji, I.E., Cheng, C.H.. "Video analytics for visual surveillance and applications: An overview and survey," in Tsihrintzis, G., Virvou, M., Sakkopoulos, E., Jain, L. (eds.), *Machine Learning Paradigms. Learning and Analytics in Intelligent Systems*, vol. 1, 2019, pp. 475–515. Springer.

24. Tokmakov, P., Alahari, K., Schmid, C. "Learning video object segmentation with visual memory," in *Proceedings of the IEEE International Conference on Computer Vision (ICCV)*, 2017, pp. 4481–4490. IEEE.

25. Rencher, A.C. *Methods of Multivariate Analysis*, 2002. Wiley-Interscience.

26. Rui, Yao, Lin, Guosheng, Xia, Shixiong, Zhao, Jiaqi, Zhou, Yong. "Video object segmentation and tracking: A survey," 1(1), 2019, 39 pages, *arXiv preprint* arXiv:1904.09172.

27. Sadaf, A., Ali, J., Irfan. "Human identification on the basis of gaits using time efficient feature extraction and temporal median background subtraction," *International Journal of Image, Graphics and Signal Processing*, 6(3), 2014, 35–42.

28. Caelles, Sergi, Maninis, Kevis-Kokitsi, Pont, Jordi -Tuset, Leal-Taixe, Laura, Cremers, Daniel, Van Gool, Luc. "One-shot video object segmentation," in *Proceedings of the IEEE Conference on Computer Vision and Pattern Recognition (CVPR)*, 2017, pp. 221–230. IEEE.

29. Stauffer, C., Grimson, W.E.L., "Adaptive background mixture models for real-time tracking," in *Proceedings of the IEEE Computer Society Conference on Computer Vision and Pattern Recognition (CVPR)*, vol. 2, 1999, pp. 246–252. IEEE.

30. Subudhi, B., Ghosh, S. "Change detection for moving object segmentation with robust background construction under Wronskian framework," *Machine Vision and Applications*, 24(4), 2013, 795–809.

31. Vecchio, S., Palazzo, D., Giordano, F., Rundo, F., Spampinato, C. "MASK-RL: Multiagent video object segmentation framework through Reinforcement Learning," *IEEE Transactions on Neural Networks and Learning Systems*, 31(12), 2020, pp. 5103–5115.

32. Verri, A., Uras, S., De Micheli, E. "Motion segmentation from optical flow," in *Proceedings of the Alvey Vision Conference*, 1989, pp. 1–6. Alvey Vision Club.

33. Zappella, Luca, Lladó, Xavier, Salvi, Joaquim. "Motion segmentation: a review," in *Proceedings of the Int. conference on Artificial Intelligence Research and Development: Proceedings of the 11th International Conference of the Catalan Association for Artificial Intelligence*, 2008, pp. 398–407. IOS Press.

7 IoMT-Based Computational Approach for Semantic Segmentation of Brain Tumour MRI Images

Sanjay Kumar and Sanjeev Kumar Singh
Information Technology Department
Galgotias College of Engineering and Technology

Naresh Kumar and Kuldeep Singh Kaswan
School of Computing Science and Technology
Galgotias University

Inderpreet Kaur
Computer Science and Engineering
Galgotias College of Engineering and Technology

Gourav Mitawa
Sobhasaria Group of Institutions

CONTENTS

DOI: 10.1201/9781003146087-9

Internet of Medical Things (IoMT) is attracting a lot of attention from the clinical scientific community. The medical devices in IoMT collect vital health-related data over the internet. Patients are given detailed supporting evidence to help them during recovery. Because of various medical equipment, attackers can change the address of devices. Certain patients suffering from illnesses like brain tumours are at risk of dying due to this. Brain tumours are caused by a mass of abnormal cells in the brain, and they can damage the brain and endanger one's life. Brain tumour diagnosis, prognosis, and treatment are all essential. The biopsy and analysis of CT scans or MRIs that are repetitive, inefficient for vast amounts of data, and enable radiologists to make assumptions are common techniques for identification. To address these issues, many software techniques have been proposed. However, there is still a great need to develop a technology that can identify a brain tumour with high specificity in a short period.

Furthermore, it is critical to select criteria that will allow predictions to attain exceptional accuracy. The brain is the most affected by tumours that grow irregularly. Early identification of such cancers greatly aids in the provision of successful therapy. The first step in diagnosing a brain tumour is to process medical images. It necessitates various imaging modalities such as computerised CT-Scan, X-ray, and magnetic resonance imaging (MRI). The primary goal of brain tumour image processing is to determine the precise size and location of the tumour in the brain. The precise size and location of the tumour aid in the identification of abnormal growth in the brain. Detection of brain tumours using MRI is a difficult endeavour even for highly trained professionals. The MRI image processing software understands how to process and segment out brain tumours. We split MRI image processing into four stages: pre-processing, picture segmentation, feature extraction, and image classification. We used various image segmentation algorithms to separate the brain tumours like seed region growing, threshold segmentation, watershed, fuzzy c-mean, histogram threshold etc. We evaluated the accuracy of various approaches and discovered that the seed region growing method outperformed with 92.5% accuracy.

7.1   INTRODUCTION

Many safety intimidations might arise with extensive medical equipment, low-power computers, and restricted safety. More specifically, IoMT management of internet equipment assists hackers in stealing patient data through the internet; hence IoT systems must also be protected. Brain tumours are the most serious threat to healthcare protection, with just 34.9% of patients surviving. Whether primary (benign) or secondary (malignant), cell proliferation in the brain is deemed abnormal, primary cancers are not malignant. They do not spread between brains, but secondary cancers are cancerous and spread throughout the body and brain. When a benign or malignant tumour develops, the skull is forced to expand, affecting the life-threatening brains. Therefore, proper prediction of brain tumours in the early stages is highly important for its diagnosis, pronouncement, and surgery. It can only be done through the application of reliable algorithms/methods on IoMT devices. Human biopsies and analysis of MRI images or CT scans are common procedures for detecting brain tumours. A pathologist examines a tiny piece of tissue under a microscope to determine the existence of a tumour. Although the anomaly is reliably revealed by biopsy, the procedure is uncomfortable for individuals. Second, if physicians opt for surgery, the specific position and percentage of the tumour must be aware of the MRI or CT scan [1]. Compared to a CT scan, an MRI image has the advantage of not containing radiation and is thus safer for human health.

Furthermore, MRI scans accurately depict malignancies. The analysis of huge amounts of human-related MRI images, on the other hand, is repetitious and inefficient, relying on the expertise of doctors and technicians. According to the findings, radiologists miss 15–27% of malignancies during screening procedures. Thus, the automated recognition of MRI pictures of brain tumours is revolutionary. Doctors can anticipate premature cell growth inside the brain by promptly detecting it and correcting the problem at an early stage [2]. Various processing techniques have been developed to automatically classify brain cancers from MRI pictures.

The brain is a component of the human body that controls the actions of the body. Brain tumours are produced by abnormal cell proliferation. Tumours are essentially uncontrolled multilane cells (tumours are uncontrolled atypical cells). A cell readily isolated from a tumour-related microcalcification, lump, and deformation. They can differ in scale, shape, and location [3]. Brain tumours are one of the leading causes of mortality in humans. Every organ in the human body has a tumour, which is an unstructured growth of tissue. It is a haphazard and wasteful accumulation of brain cells. There are about 150 distinct kinds of brain tumours; however, most brain tumours may be classified as follows: (1). noncancerous (2), pre-cancerous, (3). cancerous. A benign tumour is a non-adjacent tumour that does not develop rapidly and does not affect the surrounding healthy tissues [5]. Moles are a frequent kind of benign tumour. If they are not categorised as pre-carcinogenic tumours, they may be classified as a disease.

A malignant neoplasm is a type of tumour that worsens over time and eventually kills the affected individual; tumour cells in the skull are present and develop within a skull, known as a primary tumour [6]. Invasive brain malignancies are deadly. The tumour begins outside of the brain and progresses to the brain area known as the secondary tumour. Metastatic tumours are a prime example of a secondary tumour. The tumour is located in the brain and interferes with normal brain function. The tumour in the brain migrates to the skull, increasing brain pressure. The diagnosis of the tumour is the first stage towards healing.

Because brain pictures are placental and specialists can only view tumours, detecting a brain tumour is one of the most difficult challenges in medical image segmentation [7]. The exact location, position, and extent of the abnormal tissues are critical in brain tumour diagnosis.

"The precise position, direction, and placement of the abnormal tissues are critical in brain tumour diagnosis." Pathology analysis, pre-pressure, and integrated computer surgery can all benefit from brain MRI.

This chapter discusses the use of IoT technology to benefit healthcare systems. IoT does not have a universal definition; many references from various organisations or research groups have been used to define IoT. IoT can refer to communication between things or network (physical and logical) objects, with the internet serving as the communication network connecting them. IoT refers to items or things that actively connect with intelligent interfaces. Irregular development of a brain tumour impairs brain function and endangers life. Brain tumours are divided into two types: benign tumours and malignant tumours. Benign tumours are less dangerous than malignant tumours because malignant tumours grow fast and become life-threatening, whereas benign tumours grow gradually and consistently.

The medical image approach has been used for many years to create a visual representation of the core of a person's body for medicinal reasons [8]. MRI, CT-xcan, ultrasound, and X-ray are examples of medical imaging technology that uses a non-invasive method. Compared to other imaging modalities, MRI is primarily utilised to provide a higher resolution picture of the brain and malignant tissues. Brain tumours can therefore be identified alive using MRI scans. This study focuses on the use of imaging methods to detect brain cancers. The next section of the study covers the history of brain tumour diagnosis by image distribution. We then discuss important studies, and summarise the techniques used. The final section 5 clarifies the survey. Even though several methodologies were employed in the past studies for computational identification of brain tumours. The suggested task is best done with exact information to detect brain tumours [9]. This study, i.e. PART, was not utilised in prior trials for brain tumour detection. In terms of intricacy, PART is superior. In comparison to subsequent tests, the other preceding techniques give greater baseline performance and advanced features.

7.2 LITERATURE SURVEY

Rattan et al. proposed segmenting watersheds and using edge detection, contrast, and grayscale to identify a brain tumour. The ten information sets used to identify brain cancers by Somasundaram and Kalaiselvi were ancient, comprising standard and irregular subjects. The unwanted brain fields of the scalp, skull, and lipids are removed, and fugitive segmentation is conducted on their original muscles. Finally, complete maximum transform intensity-based tumour area detection is used. After identifying the brain tumour and removing the brain tumour field, a systematic model is proposed. To diagnose the tumour using brain MR images, a classifier called Naive Bayes is utilised. Following diagnosis, K–Mean clustering and boundary identification methods determine the brain tumour location. A genetic algorithm uses a clustering plan, area-growing technology, and intensity map [2]. The tumour characteristics, including tumour insulation in size, position, form, and intensity, were employed in an MRI picture. Watershed and threshold segmentation using this method, the image is first converted to binary format. During conversion, morphological procedures are done to separate the tumour region.

Sharma et al. developed multi-layer perception and inexperienced Bayed for tumour identification. A collection of features transferred to textural characteristics based on a GLCM is used to identify the tumour. Using morphological filters, the k-mean segmentation method is presented for identifying the tumour field. It is proposed that paradigm work be done in which the brain tumour will be automatically detected and recognised. The suggested technique consists of five stages: picture retrieval, edge identification, modified histogram clustering, pre-processing, and morphological operations. Tumours are discovered in pure white or black backgrounds following morphological functioning [4]. FP Tree — the CT scan tumour of brain pictures was created for a decision tree. The median filtering is first used as a pre-processing stage for pictures, after which texture properties are retrieved for FP Tree classification.

The OTSU Segmentation Strategy suggested the clustering density classifier for identifying brain tumours. The OTSU is an automated threshold technique that provides a single density threshold that divides pixels into two groups, the first and secondary. According to Raghavan and Damodharan, the structure provided by diverse tissues such as a tumour, grey, white, and tissue is naturally segmented [5]. Each tissue component generates segmented characteristics, which are then passed on to neural networks. Finally, the neural network is utilised to identify tumour areas. Random Forest, Brawer and Chafed are among others. Metabolic Cart costs, for example, for brain tumour classification. The vector pattern is then determined. The era of metabolic parameters and automatic tumour detection is over. It is all over. Amen et al. devised an automated approach for noise reduction; segmentation and morphology determine the tumour location. The vector to be converted to SVM is derived as the usage of various segmentation approaches. The retrieved feature set evolves depending on the segmented tumour tissue's structure, strength, and texture.

Thingspeak is the open-source IoT cloud framework, according to Noor Kareen Jumaa [1]. Bridge launched it as a supporting IoT application provider in 2010. Thing Talk is an IoT platform for adding, displaying, and evaluating live cloud data sources. Thing talk provides a quick display of data aggregated via devices and is used to prototype and test the IoT framework concept of analysis. Thing talk will combine many data sources to get more relevant results. Thing talk also assists users in operating on the environment by sending a message or activating the IP in the environment.

According to Khan Muhammad [2], current surveys, in particular, focus on the segmentation or categorisation of brain tumours utilising handcrafted techniques based on representation. As a result, there is a gap in the analysis of investigated representation-driven BTC methods. We conduct this survey on multigame CNN classification techniques with these goals in mind. We begin by separating our surveys by thoroughly analysing and assessing their merits and downsides. The second issue is addressed by creating a new section detailing existing BTC concerns and specific future study directions. A list of CNN assisted approaches used by BTC processes. The time distribution of the BTC literature on CNN is suggested.

According to Manu Gupta [3], this study proposes a novel quantitative non-invasive function for diagnosing brain tumours based on fractal texture and form data (SFTA). T2 weighted brain MRI images were utilised to identify and categorise tumour regions as LG or HG. When compared to another cutting-edge solution from the literature, our method performs significantly better. Our research enhances the usage of hybrid feature sets (texture and shape). The proposed brain tumors detection system is classified according to its accuracy. Radiologists and physicians will be able to diagnose brain tumours non-invasively using the suggested feature set.

According to Arijit Ukil [4], analytics in well-being is a difficult endeavour. However, IoT introduces a new dimension. Healthcare alternatives are convenient, dependable, and simple to use. The detection of anomalies is an essential component of healthcare checks. The portions are, in fact, irregular areas. Biomedical signal, picture, or health sample parameter data healthcare providers are a practical problem. There has been a lot of analysis focused on this subject, and the tone is meant to communicate to the brotherhood of mankind. One of the primary goals is to reduce medical errors, improve early diagnosis, and provide more accessible healthcare. It is simple to use.

According to Gunasegaram Monogram [5], there are several flaws in the check-up picture dispersion of segmentation due to variable translation and other cell characteristics. The MRI images were analysed using pre-processing, extraction, sorting, and post-processing. Classificatory algorithms such as SVM, Gadabouts, and Random Forest (RF) are utilised in segmentation. This chapter compares and contrasts three classifiers for brain tumour segmentation. This enables classification techniques to be employed based on the exact segmentation of distinct data sets. Future classifiers in production will be able to segment themselves on any database.

According to Kumar et al. [6], visual processing is used to produce an image view of the many anatomical structures of the human body. MRI scans are a distorted view of the human brain that may be used to spot tumour cells. Both help in recognising the interior anatomy of the human brain as well as checking for cell clarity. The proposed approach comprises GLCM extraction and wavelet-based area segmentation. The morphological filtering technique is sued to reduce noise. Combining the processes mentioned above reduces the complexity and efficiency of dysfunctional brain tumour cells with normal cells with enhanced accuracy.

According to Kumar, [7] some instructional lessons were provided, ranging from picture separation to the thickness of the bottom of the door. For additional cancer cell classification, this function was accomplished with a Gabor transfer across a sieve. In 2019, Alaskan proposed further approaches, such as image processing to identify malignant tumour cells. Gauss's smooth idea was utilised as a filtering target before expanding to "Fourier Fast Transformation" (FFT). Tumour analysis was carried out utilising the "NN", "Fuzzy", and tumour cell defining C condition algorithms. It takes less time to compute, but the accuracy suffers as a result. The objective of this study is to focus on tumour detection utilising imaging techniques. Chen proposes the concept of genetic tissues. Aside from this aptitude, it is suitable for diverse genetic selection.

7.3 RELATED WORK

Watershed segmentation and its usage of 2D and 3D pictures for edge detection, contrast and greyscale are used to treat brain cancers. Brain tumour diagnostic regular and pathological patients Kalaiselvi and Somasundaram [11] were utilised in the ten data sets. In this context, they showed the limbs, scalp, skull, and fats initially, and the unwanted parts in the brain are subsequently eliminated by hazy segmentation. The maximum transform-based extension is used for tumour detection. First, a structural model for brain tumour diagnosis and field extraction is suggested. To diagnosis the brain MRI tumour, a classifier is employed.

The method of Naive Bayes is included. K-mean clustering upon diagnosis to eliminate the brain tumour area, boundary identifying procedures and techniques are employed. More than 85% accuracy was achieved [12]. A colour and edge detection segmentation technique was proposed in the region of the brain tumour. Edge detection during colour segmentation using the K-mean clustering technique yields the Backpack, Gaussian operators Canny, Sobel, and Palladian. A genetic algorithm is critical for clustering, technique, and the pace of regional growth. The asymmetric map is presented in [13] to assess brain tumours. This technique employs tumour characteristics in MR pictures. The threshold and watershed are segmented by the scale of tumour isolation, location, shape, and strength [14]. The first method of converting a picture into binary representation follows that morphological transformation techniques are utilised to separate the tumour region.

Brain cancer is defined as an abnormal growth of tissue in the brain. Cases of brain tumours are on the rise today. When the shape, size, and location of a brain tumour alter, examination becomes more challenging. Brain tumours are difficult to identify in the early stages because the tumour cannot be properly quantified. However, if a brain tumour is diagnosed, proper therapy can be administered, and the patient can be cured [15]. As a result, the visible image of the inside body is made available for clinical investigation and study. Overall, MRI is a reliable and thorough technique for detecting brain cancers. Current diagnostic approaches rely on conventional human-based procedures, which raise the possibility of erroneous brain cancers. Tools and procedures for detecting tumours and their behaviour are now widely available. Brain cancers can be detected using the imaging technique. Image processing technologies transform photos into digital format and then conduct operations on them to create better and better images. This investigation will concentrate on the detection of brain cancers using imaging techniques.

Brain tumour cells in the brain contribute to tumours and brain cancers in general. Gliomas were found in the people who died. This study introduces an automatic segmentation technique for classifying gliomas using an MRI picture of the brain. As histogram and pixel strength in the segmented area are utilised to pick tumour cells, they work better than the opposite [16]. The active brain tumour detection approach improves efficiency by reducing noise and allowing for more precise segmentation procedures. According to the survey findings, an anomaly with automated ROI detection is considered a key topic of brain tumour diagnosis and study in segments and across regions of brain tumour areas.

7.4 METHODOLOGY

Brain tumours can be detected using image processing techniques based on the subsequent stages. Figure 7.1 depicts the approach utilised in the suggested analysis, diagnosis, and categorisation of brain tumours.

7.4.1 IMAGE PREPROCESSING SEGMENTATION

It is a challenging technique for the picture. Before processing an image, it is critical to remove any superfluous components. After removing unwanted artefacts, the first stage in image processing may be completed successfully [8] in Figure 7.2.

It is transforming the goshawk picture, removing the reconstruction, and removing the noise image. The most typical technique is to pre-process tumour pictures for conversion [19]. Because the image was grayscale, several approaches were employed to eliminate the extra noise filter. Non-uniformity area radio frequency (RF) produces signal amplitude variations in the homogeneity or bias area deviations due to fuzzy MRI pictures. These are as follows: inhomogeneous strength fluctuations reduce image consistency and blur, resulting in a loss of high-frequency region-specific

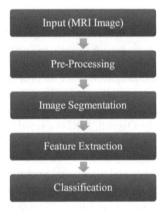

FIGURE 7.1 Steps to detected brain tumour.

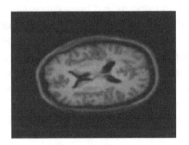 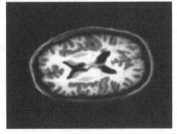

FIGURE 7.2 Original MRI image enhanced image and image enhancement [8].

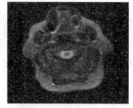
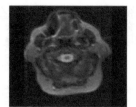

Sprinkle noise   Middle Filter image

FIGURE 7.3   Apply extremity filter [12].

information. The brain MRI volumes were first adjusted to improve tumour segmentation outcomes and the approach of extracting functionality.

7.4.2   MEDIAN FILTER IMAGES

This chapter's rising approach, no noise, filtering process is a "non-linear" method. It is used to remove the grayscale's "salt and pepper noise" [20] as shown in Figure 7.3. The convenience of the mid-protein strain works well with pepper and bran, as well as the voice of the dots. Furthermore, we have demonstrated that this impacts the usual strain's health, duration, and complexity.

7.4.3   MEAN FILTER SEGMENTS

The noise reduction strain in this method is a filter based on the standard pixel value. It will be beneficial to decrease the Gaussian clatter and the rapid comeback case on the standard filter. The sole disadvantage is that it skews boundaries and limitations.

7.4.4   WIENER FILTER SEGMENTS

Wiener filters the inverse noise reduction in the incidence domain in these approaches as well. The key format for filtering is the most efficient way to remove Wiener blur pictures. Because of his profession and because he works in the frequency domain, the pace is slow, and he is no longer suspicious.

7.4.5   IMAGE SEGMENTATION

Brain tumour volumes categorized by MRI images derived from previous research. The region of the tumour is isolated using T2-weighted MR imaging. The method is briefly discussed here. Symmetry is an important function of the brain. The brain was therefore divided into two symmetrical sections using axial axes. Then, using a subtractive approach, these half-brain areas were compared with vowels to identify tumour tissues. The non-symmetrical regions were extremely visible in the creation of pictures. Finally, it determines the largest region. There is a complete representation of all the areas. This area was subsequently recognised as a tumour location, and rest zones with a grey value of zero were used to hide the history. This method has

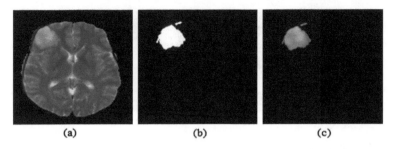

(a)   (b)   (c)

FIGURE 7.4   Pre-processed image; segmentation image.

been performed on all brain MRI slices to get a complete segmented tumour volume for any brain tumour the consequences of segmentation for one of the patients.

The picture is sometimes smaller than the portions of the image and the genealogical procedure. Similar image creation was lethal. Assign the ticket to each pixel position in the picture, like the special mark-sharing function [22] as shown in Figure 7.4. It is also important to encourage the inspection and assessment of data as a separate item.

7.4.6   THRESHOLD IMAGE SEGMENTATION

Segmentation performance was created to split the digital picture into several superpixel and fixed segments. Suggestions are only produced by simplifying the procedure that constitutes a change of image in the image, which will become more accurate and easier than a meaning resolution [23]. Hand therapy might be used to create the curve by inserting items in the pictures and the terminations. The picture is assigned a pixel by image label throughout the operation, and the elements are the same.

7.4.7   K-MEANS ALGORITHM FOR MRI

The image processing approach primarily used the K-means algorithm for frame segmentation. It is especially beneficial for large-scale images with a little change. Aside from the fact that K-means is sensitive to sample selection and the creation of fuzzy sets [14], we depict a new type of dissimilar form of segmentation in the frame.

1.   Offer a cluster value no. like k.
2.   Select k cluster centre arbitrarily
3.   The mean or core of the cluster is determined
4.   Calculate each pixel distance to each centre of the cluster
5.   When the detachment is close to the middle, go to the cluster.
6.   Go to next otherwise.
7.   Return the centre to estimate.
8.   Repeat until the core is not moving

TABLE 7.1
Different Image Segmentation Method

	Usage of MRI	Susceptible To
Doorsill process	Employ incline size to discover the possible rim Pixels [14]	firm to be second-hand meant for images with deprived difference.
Area base	Right, divide region according to towards the resemblance of property [14]	the sound might guide to excellence of last consequence
	unclear C earnings, K income plus height put technique	example assortment plus establish the blurry set, may be hard [15].

7.4.8 FEATURE EXTRACTION SEGMENTATION

The texture and form of the tumour region were important factors for determining tumour grade and malignancy degree. The function set derived is clarified in the appropriate paragraphs of the suggested analysis. Because of the brain's structure, it must be properly isolated from the brain tumour. A few readily available criteria are cautious about eliminating categories such as the organisation's size and location. The method is returned to the degree that it extracts the Edge tutor's general finding features.

7.4.9 FRACTAL-BASED TEXTURE FEATURES

The volume of the split tumour was calculated utilising the form of fractal texture based on segmentation checking. QB(r, s) multiplied by the relevant T2-weighted bias-corrected MRI slices were produced throughout the tumour mask segmentation procedure. The volume of picture output is known as QB(r, s) and is utilised for the role extraction output method. Grayscale pictures from texture characteristics "QB (r, s)" were further segregated tumour volume divided by implementation into binary images thresholding transfers sequentially. In this study, multilevel programming obtained Otsu method cut-off settings to decrease the variance infraclass picture in the input. This method has been improved, and the number of thresholds picked has been reached. These criteria must be established.

7.4.10 SHAPE MEASURES

Eccentricities and perimeters are assessed to characterise segmented tumour volume and tumour shape. However, the eccentricities were calculated as the primary ratio of big axis length for the short axis area. It has a 0 to 1 value. The perimeter is calculated by taking the width of each pair of pixels near the split field of the tumor as it approaches the border [24]. The suggested feature set comprises SFTA algorithm texture and type measurements, which were then used to classify quantities of tumour MRI as LG or Odds.

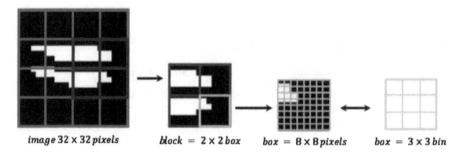

image 32 × 32 *pixels*   *block* = 2 × 2 *box*   *box* = 8 × 8 *pixels*   *box* = 3 × 3 *bin*

FIGURE 7.5   Structural design of HOG feature [17].

7.4.11 HISTOGRAM OF ORIENTED GRADIENT

In the Directed Gradient Histogram (HOG) extraction method, the following computation is performed. The picture of the pre-treated cubicle determination must be split into "3232" pixels in the initial position. Each pixel's strength is between "0" and "1." As a result, the resolution's conclusion is added to "HOG"[17]. Figure 7.5 depicts the "HOG" feature's structural architecture. As a result, the image's significance is split into "8 8" pixels known as "boxes." At this point, the will to battle has increased significantly. Each box is split into nine trays once more. In each tray, the pixel incline is utilised to construct a feature [18]. As a result, nine descriptions are easily available; this resolution directs to each item's "94" definition. The extraction of the "HOG" function creates "9 lines" in all "32 32" pixels and results in "9 9 4" characteristics in one dimension or "1 324" in:

7.4.12 CLASSIFICATION

Support Vector Machine input brain MRI categorisation is utilised in the proposed research low-grade volumes (benign) or high-grade volumes (malignant). By optimal hyperplane ejection, the input is categorised into two distinct groups in the SVM classification.

This hyperplane distinguishes between data points from one class and those from a second with the greatest reach. The training set separated the classes by the code of judgment into groups in which priors are known. From the judgment law test data set, the resulting hyperplane was used for class recognition. SVM is sufficient for the tiny sample since it can address the over-fitting problem locally, optimally and efficiently. SVM effectively maps the entry vectors in a vast space with a given dimension Kernel-specified characteristics. In this research volume of MRI input, a linear property is employed as the brain tumour in the kernel [25].

The K-fold technique was utilised for cross-validation suggested analysis to divide the data collection into tests and sets of exercises. It divides the entire data set into k mean subgroups. The grader has been tested on one of the subsets, and the remaining k-1 subsets have been trained. This is what we are referring to. Each protocol data point is duplicated k times to guarantee that it appears at least once in the evaluation data collection set of k-1 times training outcomes. Thus, feature classification is

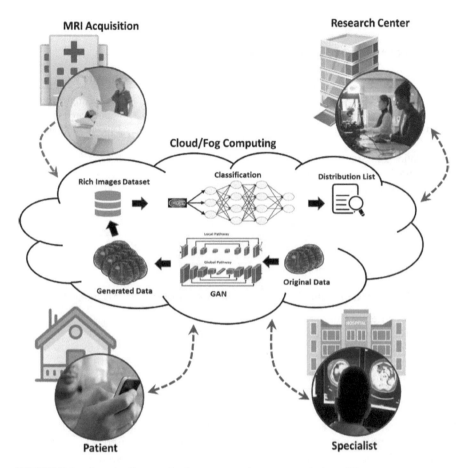

FIGURE 7.6   Generic diagram for future research recommendations [2].

extensively used in the validation of the K-fold feature classification process. It also indicates that preparation and classifier validation is taken into account for the whole dataset.

7.5   RESULT ANALYSIS

The detailed findings from future approaches for brain tumour diagnostics suggested investigation used MRI scans from the PGI 2020 confront dataset of 30 brain tumour patients as shown in Figure 7.6. Image segmentation is the most important element of image processing when detecting a brain tumour from a digital picture. Table 7.2 defines the various segmentation techniques such as accuracy plus difficulty.

In Table 7.2, three-part table advantage, computation time in sec. And flip flops used and logic to find results. The primary reason for the processing is to maintain the image edges among the perimeter detection mechanisms. Sobel combined with Gaussian, and average filters are the best option. Table 7.3 presents several edging

TABLE 7.2
Performance of Image Edge Detection

	Sobel	Robert	Prewitt
Advantages	Simplicity	Better noise suppression	Mask simpler as compared to sobal
Disadvantage	Discontinuity in edges	Not accurate results	Discontinuity in edge
Computational In Sec	0.3	0.2	0.4
Number used as Flip Flop	343	219	339
Number Used as Logic	450	322	450

TABLE 7.3
Tumour Segmentation Method

Segmentation Method	Complicity Algorithm	Accuracy %
Seed Region Grooving	10	91.5
Threshold Segmentation	8.13	91
Watershed	5.67	88
Fuzzy C-mean	5.29	85
Histogram Thresholding	7.61	81

discovery methods such as "Sobel," "Prewitt," and "Robert" in various forms, such as the calculation instance in second and the number of flip flops used.

In Table 7.3, segmentation methods and accuracy % find the seed region growing.

7.6   RESEARCH DIRECTIONS

Despite their enormous strength and effectiveness, CNN-based methods face several challenges. For example, they require a massive quantity of training data, which might be difficult, if not impossible, to get for each domain to achieve optimal accuracy on a goal problem. Furthermore, increasing the number of layers in the CNN model to enhance classification accuracy is challenging. Similarly, profound learning models are computer-consuming their underlying hardware components. Applying these models in real-world situations, particularly if an unresolved problem remains, is common in clinical practice. There are various ideas and future guidelines for community research scientists. Apply the MRI images after the tumour segmentation process and find the tumour size and location in Figure 7.7.

The pre-processed MRI picture is provided, as are the methods for K-means. The median filter was removed, and 0.05% of the salt and pepper sound was added. The K-mean method bundles the image based on those features. The performance of the five-cluster K means method is seen in Figure 7.8. In the sixth line, the tumour is eliminated.

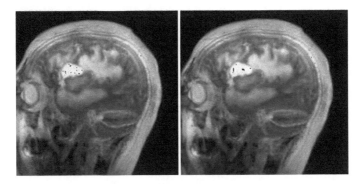

FIGURE 7.7   Steps of a brain tumour in MRI image detection.

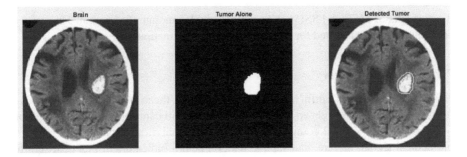

FIGURE 7.8   MRI input image

This is why we convert the RGB image to a greyscale image for a DICOM image in RGB. To add the medium filter, we utilise a 5x5 kernel with zeroes to decrease noise. Figure 7.9 depicts padded pictures.

In this organised method, several MRI scans of the brain are utilised to examine the validity of the findings. Tumours of varying structure, size, and location may be found in all three images. Following the usage of algorithms, many criteria are generally employed to assess image quality. PSNR, MSE, and SSIM are image characteristics in our study strategy that reflect the quality of our results and may also be evaluated through visualisation. For the medium filter measurement, we utilise 0.3 in image 0, 0.5 in image 1, and 0.8 in image 2. PSNR values before filter implantation range from 38.4532 to 36.2365, with a noise ratio between 0.3 and 0.5. When median filter values are applied, the outcome is not as much affected, and the picture quality stays comparable, as the visual effects are considerably uncontaminated. Before filtering, the SSIM value ranged from 5.3476 para-4 to 8.4536 para-4, and the noise ratio rose. The findings revealed a small variation in values, ranging from 6.5287 para-4 to 5.234 para 3, immediately after the filtration results. The MSE values indicate the variance. We compute the same parameter bordered by the MRI image and the cross rim detector to comprehend the hybrid edge detector output. PSNR readings for salt and pepper noise range from 36.345 to 34.213 this time. Compared to the original picture,

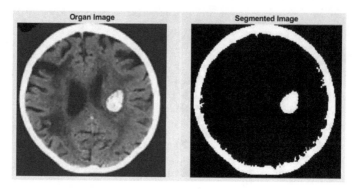

FIGURE 7.9   Padded images.

the concepts of MSE and SSIM show a comparable amount of variation. The created approach is well renowned for maintaining image perfection.

7.7   CONCLUSION

Healthcare analytics is a difficult endeavour. However, the arrival of IoT raises the bar for developing realistic, cheap, and simple-to-use healthcare solutions. The detection of anomalies is a critical component of healthcare analytics. Anomaly areas are the biomedical signal, picture, and sample data on health indicators of practical significance to medical practitioners. This is a significant subject of research, and the human brotherhood has to give a lot. One of the top goals will be to minimise diagnostic error, enhance early infection detection, improve prognostics, and deliver inexpensive and simple-to-use healthcare. The primary goal of brain tumour image processing is to determine the precise size and location of the tumour in the brain. We utilise medical imaging in this study to find the most accurate and relevant sequence imagery with the least degree of inaccuracy. Because of the intricacy of brain scans, identifying a tumour using a brain MRI picture is a difficult process. The tumour understands how to communicate with a variety of cutting-edge imaging treatments. The technique is the same when utilising MRI brain pictures that four-part processing can detach; just an image and extract partition representation is used. The median filter is frequently used in a variety of arts for filtering. It is easier to get rid of power, pepper, and scream; what are the main advantages of pressure? As opposed to the Gaussian strain, the non-linear strain of the filter is the filter that retains the edges. Furthermore, these are low-pass filters with a role in sequence determination that is misdirected on the boundaries that will be excited and unclear.

REFERENCES

1.   Ukil, Arijit, Bandyoapdhyay, Soma, Puri, Chetanya, Pal, Arpan. "IoT healthcare analytics: The importance of anomaly detection," in *2016 IEEE 30th International Conference on Advanced Information Networking and Applications (AINA)*, 2016, pp. 994–997. IEEE.

2. Khan, Muhammad, Khan, Salman, Del Ser, Javier, de Albuquerque, Victor Hugo C. "Deep learning for multigrade brain tumour classification in smart healthcare systems: A prospective survey," *IEEE Transactions on Neural Networks and Learning Systems*, 32(2), 2020, 507–522.

3. Manogaran, Gunasekaran, Shakeel, P. Mohamed, Hassanein, Azza S., Kumar, Priyan Malarvizhi, Babu, Gokulnath Chandra. "Machine learning approach-based gamma distribution for brain tumour detection and data sample imbalance analysis." *IEEE Access*, 7, 2018, 12–19.

4. Jumaa, Noor Kareem, Mohamad, Auday A.H., Majeed, Sameer Hameed. "Internet of things mathematical approach for detecting brain tumour," *International Journal of Engineering & Technology*, 7(4), 2018, 2779–2783.

5. Kumar, Sanjay, Negi, Ashish, Singh, J.N. "Semantic segmentation using deep learning for brain tumour MRI via fully convolution neural networks," in *Information and Communication Technology for Intelligent Systems*, 2019, pp. 11–19. Springer.

6. Kumar, Sanjay, Negi, Ashish, Singh, J.N., Verma, Himanshu. "A deep learning for brain tumour MRI images semantic segmentation using FCN," in *2018 4th International Conference on Computing Communication and Automation (ICCCA)* , 2018, pp. 1–4. IEEE.

7. Kumar, Sanjay, Singh, Jitender Nath and Nagi, Ashish. "An Amalgam Method efficient for Finding of Cancer Gene using CSC from Micro Array Data," *International Journal on Emerging Technologies*, 11(3), 2020, 207–211.

8. Kabade, Rohit S., Gaikwad, M.S. "Segmentation of brain tumour and its area calculation in brain MR images using K-mean clustering and fuzzy C-mean algorithm," *International Journal of Computer Science & Engineering Technology*, 4(05), 2013, 524–531.

9. Alwazzan, Mohammed J., Ismael, Mohammed A., Hussain, Moaid. "Brain tumour isolation in MRI images based on statistical properties and morphological process techniques," *Journal of Physics: Conference Series*, 1279(1) , 2019, p. 012018.

10. Maharjan, Sunil, Alsadoon, Abeer, Prasad, P.W.C., Al-Dalain, Thair, Alsadoon, Omar Hisham. "A novel enhanced softmax loss function for brain tumour detection using deep learning," *Journal of Neuroscience Methods*, 330, 2020, 108520.

11. Wadhwa, Anjali, Bhardwaj, Anuj, Verma, Vivek Singh. "A review on brain tumour segmentation of MRI images," *Magnetic Resonance Imaging*, 61, 2019, 247–259.

12. Kollem, Sreedhar, Reddy, Katta Rama Linga, Rao, Duggirala Srinivasa. "A review of image denoising and segmentation methods based on medical images," *International Journal of Machine Learning and Computing*, 9(3), 2019, 288–295.

13. Sazzad, T.M. Shahriar, Ahmmed, K.M. Tanzibul, Ul Hoque, Misbah, Rahman, Mahmuda. "Development of automated brain tumour identification using MRI images," in *2019 International Conference on Electrical, Computer and Communication Engineering (ECCE)*, 2019, pp. 1–4. IEEE.

14. Al-Absi, Hamada R.H., Abdullah, Azween, Hassan, Mahamat Issa. "Soft computing in medical diagnostic applications: A short review," in *2011 National Postgraduate Conference*, 2011, pp. 1–5. IEEE.

15. Kaya, Duygu, Turk, Mustafa. "LabVIEW based robust cascade predictive model for evaluating cancer prognosis," *Physica A: Statistical Mechanics and its Applications*, 549, 2020, 123978.

16. Sellami, Ali, Hwang, Heasoo. "A robust deep convolutional neural network with batch-weighted loss for heartbeat classification," *Expert Systems with Applications*, 122, 2019, 75–84.

17. Maltarollo, Vinicius Goncalves, Kronenberger, Thales, Espinoza, Gabriel Zarzana, Oliveira, Patricia Rufino, Honorio, Kathia Maria. "Advances with support vector machines for novel drug discovery," *Expert Opinion on Drug Discovery*, 14(1), 2019, 23–33.

18. Sharif, Muhammad Irfan, Li, Jian Ping, Naz, Javeria, Rashid, Iqra. "A comprehensive review on multi-organs tumour detection based on machine learning," *Pattern Recognition Letters*, 131, 2020, 30–37.

19. Wadhwa, Anjali, Bhardwaj, Anuj, Verma, Vivek Singh. "A review on brain tumour segmentation of MRI images," *Magnetic resonance imaging*, 61, 2019, 247–259.

20. Kumar, Sanjay, Negi, Ashish, Singh, J.N., Gaurav, Amit. "Brain tumour segmentation and classification using MRI images via fully convolution neural networks," in *2018 International Conference on Advances in Computing, Communication Control and Networking (ICACCCN)*, 2018, pp. 1178–1181. IEEE.

21. Gomathi, Parkash, Baskar, Sunil, Shakeel, Mohamed Paven. "Numerical function optimisation in brain tumour regions using reconfigured multi-objective bat optimisation algorithm," *Journal of Medical Imaging and Health Informatics*, 9(3), 2019, 482–489.

22. Khan, Hikmat, Shah, Pir Masoom, Shah, Munam Ali, ul Islam, Saif, Rodrigues, Joel J.P.C. "Cascading handcrafted features and convolutional neural network for IoT-enabled brain tumour segmentation," *Computer Communications*, 153, 2020: 196–207.

23. Chen, Hao, Qin, Zhiguang, Yi, Ding, Lan, Tian, Qin, Zhen. "Brain tumour segmentation with deep convolutional symmetric neural network." *Neurocomputing*, 392, 2020, 305–313.

24. Ganesan, P., Sathish, B.S., Elamaran, V., Murugesan, R. "Brain Tumour Segmentation and Measurement Based on Threshold and Support Vector Machine Classifier," *Research Journal of Pharmacy and Technology*, 13(6), 2020, 2573–2577.

25. Işın, Ali, Direkoğlu, Cem, Şah, Melike. "Review of MRI-based brain tumour image segmentation using deep learning methods," *Procedia Computer Science*, 102, 2016, 317–324.

26. Usman, Khalid, Rajpoot, Kashif. "Brain tumour classification from multi-modality MRI using wavelets and machine learning," *Pattern Analysis and Applications*, 20(3), 2017, 871–881.

27. Xiao, Zhe, Huang, Ruohan, Ding, Yi, Lan, Tian, Dong, RongFeng, Qin, Zhiguang, Zhang, Xinjie, Wang, Wei. "A deep learning-based segmentation method for brain tumour in MR images," in *2016 IEEE 6th International Conference on Computational Advances in Bio and Medical Sciences (ICCABS)* , 2016, pp. 1–6. IEEE.

28. Havaei, Mohammad, Davy, Axel, Warde-Farley, David, Biard, Antoine, Courville, Aaron, Bengio, Yoshua, Pal, Chris, Jodoin, Pierre-Marc, Larochelle, Hugo. "Brain tumour segmentation with deep neural networks," *Medical Image Analysis*, 35, 2017, 18–31.

29. Shanker, Ravi, Bhattacharya, Mahua. "Brain tumour segmentation of normal and pathological tissues using K-mean clustering with fuzzy C-mean clustering," in *European Congress on Computational Methods in Applied Sciences and Engineering*, 2017, pp. 286–296. Springer.

30. Roy, Sudipta, Bhattacharyya, Debnath, Bandyopadhyay, Samir Kumar, Kim, Tai-Hoon. "Heterogeneity of human brain tumour with lesion identification, localisation, and analysis from MRI," *Informatics in Medicine Unlocked*, 13, 2018, 139–150.

Unit 3

IoT-Based Systems for Healthcare Industries
Opportunities and Challenges

8 Internet of Medical Things

Smart Healthcare Monitoring Systems and Their Potential Implementations

Safaa N. Saud Al-Humairi, Asif Iqbal Hajamydeen, and Husniza Razalli
Faculty of Information Sciences and Engineering
Management and Science University

CONTENTS

DOI: 10.1201/9781003146087-11

Smart healthcare is rapidly transforming from a traditional model based on hospitals' demand to a global patient-centred approach. Many technological advancements have facilitated this rapid transition in vertical healthcare. Recently, the assistance offered by intelligent medical instruments and the Internet of Things (IoT) has transformed healthcare approaches worldwide. In this context, the cloud and IoT architectures are often used to enable smart healthcare systems to support real-time applications through artificial intelligence processing and analysis of the massive amounts of data created by wearable sensor networks. However, response and cloud-based systems and security and privacy are critical, preventing the Internet of Medical Things (IoMT) devices and architectures from providing a safe and effective solution to the user. This chapter briefly discusses a breakthrough for IoT-based medical technology and explores the state-of-the-art networking architectures, industrial applications, and developments in IoT-based solutions. It also discusses features in the protection and privacy of IoT inclusively with medical security requirements. Furthermore, this chapter also introduces an intelligent collaborative security model to reduce safety risks, given the current crisis of Covid-19. It also deliberates various developments and the extensive usage of big data and artificial intelligence in medical services.

8.1   BACKGROUND TO IOMT

IoT describes the network of physical objects, "things" that are embedded with sensors, software, and other technologies to connect and exchange data with other devices and systems over the internet. IoT is characterised as a dynamic and self-configured network using interoperable communication protocols, media, and standards [1, 2] for physical and virtual objects.

The objects include even household lights to different domestic appliances, vehicles, and all devices around us to communicate with other machines or devices. IoT enables devices or objects that can communicate over the internet by using physical devices, sensors, microcontrollers, and network connectivity to capture and share data between these objects. Each computer has a unique UID, making communication simple, such as machine-to-machine (M2M) communication, to accumulate real-time data consistently. Massive data from computers worldwide are processed in the cloud, improving machine productivity and intelligence. IoT creates intelligent objects constituting the building blocks for enhancing the universal frameworks of cyber-physical intelligence. They are intended for millions of physical items or objects with various sensors and actuators linked via the internet through various access networks enabled by various technologies, such as wireless sensor networks (WSN), RFID, real-time and web services [3]. Therefore, IoT may be considered a new IT (ICT) variant of the ICT and has also created a new challenge in the medical sector, the IoMT, ranging from smart devices to innovative cities. Increasing the quality of life and reducing medical costs delivers significant benefits for people's well-being. As shown in Figure 8.1, the critical elements are wireless sensors, which can be used to track the health status through the communication technologies of patients to send information to caregivers.

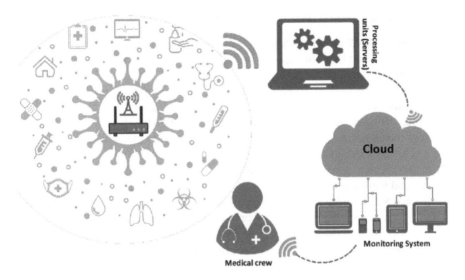

FIGURE 8.1 IoMT system architecture.

IoMT can be used for clinical decisions due to artificial intelligence, telemedicine, and sensor technology developments. Human decisions, assisted by virtual assistants, are already used by hospitals in radiology and can gather the secret factors of extensive healthcare data using sophisticated algorithms such as deep learning [4, 5]. IoMT may also equip additional self-correction skills to boost preciseness after feedback. Digital assistants can keep doctors updated by presenting new knowledge for proper patient treatment from various posts, journals, and clinical practices [6]. IoMT can be used to continuously track patients' lives, generate alarms, and sometimes take the appropriate precautions under changing health conditions.

Artificial intelligence-supported IoMT devices can regularly track human health. Smart robots, smart homes, and virtual assistants assist the elderly and disabled people with the help they need. Epidemic diseases can be followed and avoided by integrating the data collected with the IoMT sensors with the health system's information. Smart systems empower authorities during emergencies and deliver practical assistance for people and take appropriate action promptly.

IoMT works collaboratively to provide the best healthcare facilities effectively and healthily with input components like biosensors, communication modules, and users. IoMT technology's support is a significant factor in developing ecosystems, especially those using remote monitoring systems, like self-care and early diagnosis [7]. A remote monitoring system is essential if the data collected through bio-sensors are processed and analysed on a real-time basis. Data sharing between these devices requires protected mechanisms and technologies of communication. Data leakage and theft of information are significant issues if such devices are not adequately protected.

8.2   GENERAL ARCHITECTURE OF IOT

IoT, one of the most critical technologies of the future, has gained much attention for more than a decade [8]. Although the concept is widely used and the technology has been applied, it is indistinct what IoT encompasses [9]. Ashton and Brock from the Massachusetts Institute of Technology initiated IoT by founding an Auto-ID Center to clarify the Auto-ID reflection on any form of technology to track the objects while travelling between sites [10]. Since the inception of IoT, scholars have suggested different meanings. Lee et al. [8] describe IoT as a worldwide network of computers and machinery that can communicate with each other, often called the Internet of All. Yin et al. [10] also note that IoT consists of a collection from which several networked devices and appliances facilitate interaction and communication. IoT is described by Bouhai and Saleh [11] as a network that continuously extends and connects traditional material objects with the internet. Farahani et al. [12] have established the IoT's eco-system side via a network, which permits connecting, collecting, and exchanging information to continually develop an ecosystem that integrates the functionality of the hardware, software, and physical objects.

For businesses to adapt their business models entirely, it has been reported that the disruptive strength of IoT brings new products and technological solutions for the current needs [13]. Recently, IoT represents intelligent connected devices with enhanced data-generation capabilities. It includes physical components such as a product's mechanical and electrical parts, smart features such as sensors, controls and storage of data, ports, antennas, and wire/wireless connections. Three ways to link IoT products are (1) one-by-one connection of a single product with a user, (2) connection of a central device to several products concurrently, or (3) multiple connections of products to external data sources [14, 15].

The growth in the use of health technology in the administration of patients' health is called digital health [16], which means that the use of these technologies improves patient health. Lyawa et al. [16] describe digital health as a change in healthcare providers methods in using ICT to track and enhance patient safety and permit them to manage their health. A common term for digital health provides a diverse set of definitions, including eHealth, mHealth, and connected health with the internet [17]. Although eHealth denotes the internet and network technologies related to health aids, mobile applications represented by mHealth are also utilised for healthcare assistance [16].

Digital health has introduced an extensive variety of innovations to healthcare [18]. The new ways to monitor, calculate, and view a human body for healthcare are supported by mobile applications, tablets, platforms, and websites. In addition, innovations like health sensors, ECG-connected smartphones, telemedicine, and genome sequencing are increasingly disruptive. These advances are also needed to lead to more value-based healthcare, contribute to clinical assessment, and enable patients to receive treatment. Technologies brand healthcare and stimulate the patients in contributing to performance and satisfaction [19]. IoT-based healthcare solutions are among these modernisations to increase access to healthcare and boost quality while reducing costs.

Healthcare is one of the sectors that have adopted IoT applications over the last few years. Healthcare integrated services integrate various treatment operations such as remote observation, diagnosis, and online surgery [10] and gather data from patients, equipment, and materials through monitoring and tracking [20]. This cross-sectional IoT application has paved the way for the Internet of Health Stuff [21] to IoMT. IoMT is referred to as "the connectivity of medical devices via an online system like web-cloud, which frequently encompasses machine-to-machine (M2M) communications," as described by Basatneh et al. [22]. IoMT encapsulates software, healthcare, systems, and medical device-based infrastructure [21].

Although IoMT is still in its infancy [22], remote control systems such as wearables have increased interest in recent years. A growing number of devices on the market have become available [23]. The networked sensors of IoMT are integrated into or used to collect data, demonstrating well-being data about the patient's environment. Sensors can detect signs and biometric data used in a previous state/situation to identify health conditions. Besides, portable sensors offer consumers updated information on their well-being and deliver healthcare professionals real-time information [24]. The solution for clarification is provided in Figure 8.2, as the analytical study unit for this research offers remote monitoring solutions. While solutions take various forms, sensors, data storage, central repositories, and diagnostic applications are typically components [25].

Research exposes the ability of IoT technologies to concurrently and dramatically enhance healthcare professionals' and patients' performance and well-being [20]. A study of IoMT research has centred primarily on three points, identifying the technology [26], opportunities, and how it can be used [22]. It details the research on the issues with security and privacy [27]. Opportunities and threats have been illustrated as part of the research community on IoMT [26].

The medical internet advances and expands healthcare facilities in different ways. Farahani et al. [12] clarify IoMT in providing a holistic solution to public needs. IoMT combines various technologies to function seamlessly and offers the potential for user-friendly content or service personalisation. The patient can be tracked for life with IoMT and thus be fully viewed in the long term [28]. IoMT also aims

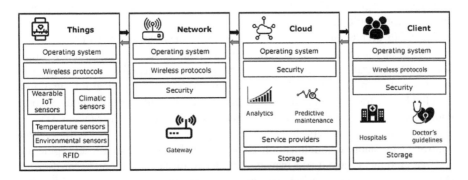

FIGURE 8.2 Architecture for IoMT monitoring; adapted from [26].

to minimise healthcare expenses by enabling patients to track their health and only consult physicians if the status falls below the recommendation. As stated by Gulraiz et al. [29], IoMT increases the system's simplicity and ease of use, thus improving healthcare efficiency and reducing costs. Furthermore, doctors can contribute more by accessing real-time health status information, thereby depending on IT healthcare services to track many patients. Healthcare practitioners and patients need health status information at any time and, eventually, IoMT will provide availability and accessibility on such information irrespective of location. Lindman and Saarikko [9] address the main solutions that can increase patient safety by providing information to medical professionals if they need help. In a nutshell, IoMT offers the ability to provide higher quality healthcare at reduced costs and ultimately provides a longer lifespan.

8.3   EHEALTH SOLUTION USING IOT

The facility of health services under the umbrella of eHealth requires a broad implementation of ICTs. Surveys and various implementations are explored about identifying their primary building blocks as a basis for the dissertation's proposed telemonitoring prototype. Sawand et al. [30] addressed eHealth monitoring system performance by explaining the entire life cycle and identifying the primary factors involved in the operation. They offer patient data collection as an integral basis for robust, efficient, and reliable health surveillance. This system addresses safety risks to eHealth surveillance systems and recognises obstacles in the design to deliver high-quality and healthy patient-centred surveillance systems with a few possible solutions. E-Healthcare is a promising area of application that can enhance the quality of medical care while creating a high degree of technological integration among IoT, cloud computing and wireless body area networks (WBANs). WBAN is now the main provider of in-patient and remote monitoring and is expected to surpass the existing status of the healthcare and real-time monitoring market. Besides this, computation or storage outsourcing is simpler due to the awareness of the benefits of the cloud computing platform for the cloud service providers (CSPs) and customers. The authors say that tracking patient-centred health plays a crucial role in the engineering hardware description (EHD), as health practices are transferred to user-friendly environments from traditional clinical settings.

The CSPs architecture, shown in Figure 8.3, is taken up by Sawand et al. [30]. It consists of an interconnected network of heterogeneous sensors rather than a Simple Station (BS) overall system. The controller creates a connection to a PS/Smartphone, which, on the other hand, regularly or on-demand transmits medical information to the cloud (e.g., transmission powered by events). PS is used primarily by the medical data aggrandization application, which interfaces between heterogeneous sensors, end-users and cloud servers. It enables heterogeneous sensors to be configured and controlled as stable communication channels; such a device can track epidemics in large amounts to avoid and manage productive diseases in mobile crowdsensing (MCS) or participatory sensing. The authors define and position several obligations for patients and physicians, and healthcare workers, whose job is to access different medical datasets in the sludge simpler for physicians. In achieving the objective of the

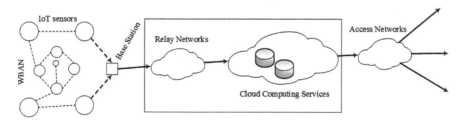

FIGURE 8.3   The CPS system architecture for remote monitoring [30].

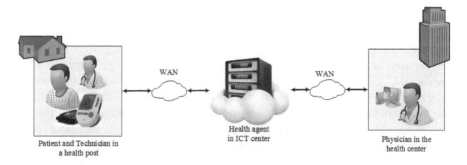

FIGURE 8.4   A telemonitoring scenario [31].

telemonitoring system, the use of human agents to transmit information, particularly in emergencies, is a serious disadvantage. This system can be redefined to automate the maximum processing allocated to MSPs, such as the transmission to a designated physician, specialist physician, and or emergency centre of troubling medical data of specific patients.

The approach to remote monitoring and telemedicine in developing countries are explored by Juha Puustjarvi and Leena Puustjarvi [31]. They claim that many of the population live in rural areas in developed countries, while many trained doctors live in urban centres. Therefore, they discuss that those trained physicians' services can be extended to remote and inaccessible regions using telemedicine. The use of relatively inexpensive equipment and targeting those regions of high doctor-to-patient ratios will make this easier. The authors' approach has stressed using information therapy to carry out automated remote monitoring [32]. As shown in Figure 8.4, medical employees can easily transfer trivial tasks to a health office tool. They submit that these solutions should focus on patients and thus underline the importance of the ability of patients to recognise and use their health records with minimal assistance. The key to their work recognises the use of knowledge therapy and qualified stakeholders' need to use those strategies effectively. Furthermore, they note that these systems' importance is never thoroughly utilised and understood without proper training.

The Alahmadi and Soh [33] implementation of eHealth Management Systems follows a different approach showing that availability, efficiency, and quality of service are crucial to any eHealth monitoring system (QoS). Its work is based on a mobile device architecture consisting of three decision layers that integrate different features for patients and medical personnel, such as knowledge, agility, reliability, scalability, and flexibility. A decentralised approach has been proposed with three layers of the processing and analysis of data, tablets, PCs and the main server. The work on WSNs was developed, and the need to focus on patients was highlighted. If a patient is not close to the PC, the smartphone is used to gather vital signals from the sensors. The server serves as the primary research centre and database interface for the diagnostic use of historical data. It also serves as the initiator of stakeholder contact. Although its proposed architecture allows a mobile environment to track and provide input based on time, the PC seems dispensable.

Archer et al. [34] introduce a predictive health evaluation approach to eHealth record system design for elderly treatment. This focuses on integrating health information with the data for elderly care from environmental sensors. To improve healthcare and independent living as people grow older, they argue that environmental sensors need to be utilised beyond the critical sign data. They argued that the added environment sensor background gave physicians great tools/resources and reduced caregivers' workload. The authors also analysed the role played in the execution of live assistants via supplementary functions, including daily alerts, rapid alarms, and real-time healthcare. It can provide doctors with additional features, including setting sensor thresholds and transmitting unique messages to patients remotely. Their works also bring families and friends closest to patients outside of the hospital into the monitoring equation.

Mukherjee et al. [35] deliberate that television surveillance solutions will allow parents to supervise their children and provide emergency response services (ERS). The vision, middleware, APIs and application layers and services as the blocks of such an architecture are defined in Figure 8.5. It can use a laptop or handheld device to integrate and process data from wearable sensor arrays (smartphones). These aggregated data are related to sensor data installed and transmitted to cloud-hosted servers. Because of the easy access by stakeholders and the processing offered to predict possible issues, the authors believe the cloud servers were used for data storage. In this application, the smartphone feature is the compilation, processing, and transfer of data from the available sensors to the cloud server. Both the API

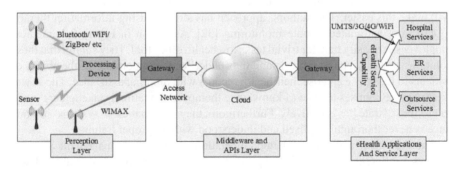

FIGURE 8.5   Illustration of the eHealth monitoring architecture [35].

provider and the app and services for the cloud server feature. It performs crucial procedures such as an emergency response analysis and lets the doctor provide on-the-spot consultation. This tremendous dependency on the cloud server means that the available internet connections cannot always be guaranteed. The architecture shown in Figure 8.5 consists of three elements. The authors also conclude that with a more significant number of sensors or better sensor and treatment capabilities, the precision of the obtained data and the responsiveness to an immediate emergency could be improved.

The use of background and location sensors for monitoring patients is extended by Szakacs-Simon et al. [36]. This device was fulfilled by an Android application for improved coverage of the control facilities and the monitoring of patients in real time. A smartphone's function extends from the transmission of vital data signs to a tracking system. The authors also stress the use of mobile features, such as sending SMS notifications. These allow patients even outside their homes to be tracked in real time. This is the first study to integrate a telemonitoring approach using reverse geocoding. Another distinguishing strategy is intrinsic mobile phone features (real-time data transfer, GPS, SMS). As shown in Figure 8.6, the authors use three components (RMD, mobile, and central server) to apply their process. The higher the participation esteem then the more the information close to the bunch focus. The summation of participation of every datum point ought to be equivalent to one. The use of the intelligent node of wireless communication (W-iPCN) is assumed to be a set of sensors because of its value for adding significance to data on vital

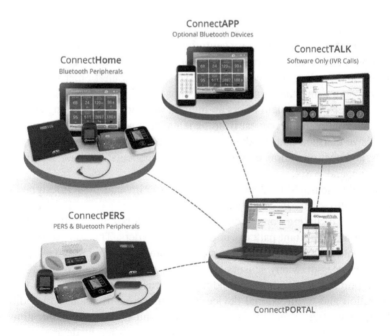

FIGURE 8.6 Component's architecture.

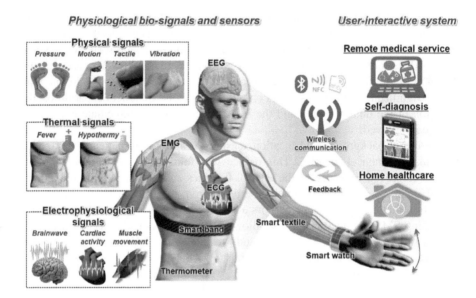

FIGURE 8.7   Implementation of a combination of multiple sensors [37].

signs (medical sensors and environmental sensors) [37]. Figure 8.7 shows the relation between the different components. The W-iPCN screens and transmits data to a
remote server.

The wireless protocol functionality in the W-iPCN can also be reconfigured and
adapted to various kinds of protocols. The smartphone is used to establish the hospital data transfer in real time to a central computer server system for track records
and remote access. In the event of an emergency, through speech messages, text
messages, and sending notified remote servers that can alert other stakeholders/dis-
tance networks using the communication capacity of the smartphones. The remote
database server of the system offers an Internet interface for collecting and accessing
patient information upon request from patients, doctors, and registered persons. The
authors have clarified that the device supports users who need ongoing monitoring,
analysis, and post-operation, comprising four components: database server, W-iPCN,
smartphone, and WSN.

A wearable sensors-based overview of an experimental model designed to track
patients' health status is described by Butca et al. [38] to evaluate and compare
various signs, including voice, body temperature, carbon monoxide level and heart
rate, which are important patterns in different disorders. The authors stated that the
aggregate data must be transmitted to a cloud storage system through a local gateway
by a microprocessor. Many sensors are used for body temperature and air moisture.
The local portal accepts processed and indexed sensor data, provides data to monitor,
configuration and bi-directional device data sensing environments. In addition, the
local gateway offers user information security and allows communication across
standardised network protocols and interfaces with different devices. The author

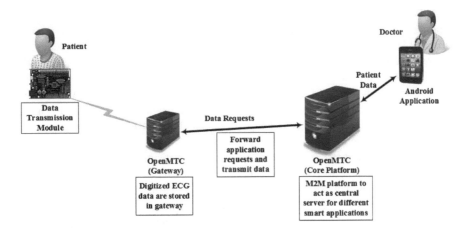

FIGURE 8.8 The ECG monitoring system architecture [39].

argues that cloud computing is highly scalable, cost-effective and multifaceted, even with unreliable network performance, apps and applications.

Conclusively, Suryani et al. [39] constructed a way to track heart activity using middleware (an OpenMTC platform). Middleware is used in the framework provided to permit data transmission between multiple points (ECG) and smartphones. It has an ECG device, an Android app for middleware access, patient information reception and ECG output displays. In the middleware configuration, the ECG measures data to be stored and viewed with an android device. Figure 8.8 displays the architecture of the monitoring system.

8.3.1 MONITORING DEVICES

Smart healthcare technology in today's healthcare system is one of the most innovative. The patient-generated data can be submitted to electronic devices and health records using intelligent wearable devices, empowering physicians to track patient action in real-time, reducing healthcare costs. In the healthcare sector, there are many wired intelligent devices. Generally, the patients consult the doctor on their respiratory issues and sugar levels. Currently, patients may use wearable apps, phone apps, and sensors at home to collect information and direct the data to a healthcare provider permitting the medical practitioner to track the patient and provide the right prescription if an issue arises

Fleetcher et al. [40] addressed the production and supply of affective computing of a sensing system based on the 802.15.4 wireless standard. It claims that developing new technologies to sensor autonomous knowledge in new health and medical research fields is possible by developing low-power radio electronics and wireless protocols. It also demonstrates that new sensors collect data comparable to data collected from the conventional electrodermal activity and heart rate sensors, though not traditional in positioning and design. ZigBee was chosen as an ideal designer as the radio hardware is unfriendly. This system includes a low-cost, comfortable, and durable sensor module built, providing the needed capacities for effective sensing. Luxner [41] has developed an option for a BP-controlled mobile device to the expensive ambulatory blood pressure monitor (ABPMs). The user will display a BP (Made by Amron) monitor via an Arduino board and, therefore, the readings will be extracted from the stand and sent to a mobile phone via Bluetooth. The authors focused on linking and transmitting the readings to a data server. It is said that a few functionalities such as read storage and view display from ABPM to the mobile application will make the monitor smaller, more convenient, and potentially cheaper. The exertion only showed the ability to obtain data at the displayed price. However, the authors were also able to accomplish the objective of what was called "hacking" in proprietary devices. The author acknowledges, however, that deploying the system in real life will be difficult. It maintains that a unique or qualified circuit board must be compacted with the design and related installations so that the system proposed does not operate on the ground.

Surveillance systems are presented in the development and implementation. The tech industry played a major role in developing these products. Withing's, a part of Nokia, has, for instance, produced a large number of wearables and measurement instruments (e.g., smartwatches, Withing's Pulse, and Withing's BP monitor) [42]. There has been much work in the fitness sector in developing wearables, particularly cardiac monitoring systems. Examples include chest-binding heart rate monitors (HRMs) such as Zephyr HxM BT [43], Myzone-MZ-3 [44], and Garmin's HRM-Tri [45]. Employers commonly use these for determining the health of employees. Activities include walking, bicycling, hiking, playing, sleeping, and much more for observing.

8.3.2   HELO WRISTBAND

Helo wristband is an in-patient real-time health monitor, round the clock with disease prediction. It can track exercise, emotions, blood pressure, heart rate, and electromagnetic diagnostics (ECG) every single moment in the body. This bracelet has active sensors that can feel the temperature of the body. The report will be sent to family members, and they can automatically monitor the patient's GPS location if a problem arises [46].

8.3.3   WIRELESS BLOOD PRESSURE MONITOR

This instrument measures the patient's blood pressure and a wireless monitor with a wireless link through Bluetooth to a smartphone app. The patient is tracked in real time and informed of the proper treatment [47].

8.3.4   ALIVECOR HEART MONITOR

An intelligent sensor that connects to the phone box wirelessly with the smartphone application and collects the ECG recording is called AliveCor Heart Monitor. The ECG level varies; the direct contact is established with the assigned doctor [48].

8.3.5 Cloud Computing

The value of web applications cannot be overemphasised in telemonitoring systems, and the intelligent medical server is positioned as the backbone of the intelligent medical server. In addition to a user-to-data interface, they propose patient-specific thresholds learned from historical data and preserve the information in a central database. In addition to concurrent access by multiple stakeholders, Kakria et al. [49] introduced web applications. This system is achieved by using the Laravel PHP platform to implement web interfaces. The web application interface reflects the same approach in web service design using Apache Tomcat [50], Java web server [51] and MySQL database [52]. The web server uses the web page to manage HTTP requests sent to the Java servers and Java Server Pages (JSP) web container that handles the Java server runtime environment. Consequently, the Java execution results are returned as HTTP responses to the client.

As previously stated, the web is supported fast that displays only vital signage, interacts, and displays its services through interfaces to the rest of the system. A robust application should, however, be built to maximise the benefits of these tools. Yii has a framework, an example for implementing a powerful web application [53]. These web apps can be configured and made pervasive with the advent of cloud computing. The NIST [54] defines cloud computing as a model for fast management and/or SP participation, enabling sharing common configurable computing resources (e.g., networks, servers, storing applications, and services). Cloud computing also provides a platform to deploy web and other information efficiently (e.g., the M2M middleware).

8.3.6 End-User's Applications

Using a mobile-optimised application or web browsers using any device, SDKs like Android, iOS, or Windows Phone SDK can create customised applications. The key factor is the target market, although other factors influence the choice of an SDK. Wang et al. [55] address the usage of Android mobile platforms in remote control systems, stating Android mobile systems dramatically decrease investment in healthcare facilities and make healthcare safer and more practical than traditional healthcare, among many other aspects. They have also realised the importance of inherent functions and tools that feature high quality visual (GUI) features and mobile Android platforms such as SQLite (lightweight) databases. Due to Android mobile networking capacities, the authors acknowledge that access to other networks, including cloud providers, middleware, and servers, is simplified.

In addition, leading companies, such as Health and Google Fit, have developed various applications to monitor vital signs. Health is an easy-to-use application developed with the iOS SDK by Apple Inc. It consolidates health information from iPhones, Apple Watch, and some prominent third-party apps that enable users to track progress in an activity in a convenient location. The four aspects of good health (as much as you move), sleep (as well as rest) and concentration (as well as rest), and food have been identified as activities (as well as your food). However, it does not completely automate stakeholder correspondence and sends data to proprietary servers.

Google Fit [56] is an Android operating system (Android SDK) health-tracking software created by Google Fits, enabling users to monitor behaviours easily by automatically tracking them with Google Fit on an Android phone or Android Watch. It is also an online portal with activity data such as speed, rhythm, paths, lifting that can be viewed through the phone, tablet, site, or Android Wear watch from anywhere. Its goal is a fitness application. It sends data like health to proprietary servers and does not completely automate communication with stakeholders. Although such applications and monitoring devices are widely used, especially in the fitness sector, automation is limited, particularly if stakeholders are informed; central servers such as Apple, Google, Omron and Withing's are typically operated by manufacturers and thus prevent users from using them in their entirety.

8.4 SECURITY AND PRIVACY ISSUES OF IOMT

IOT's primary security and privacy concerns are authentication, identification, and system heterogeneity. Besides, convergence, scalability, connectivity and ethics processes, business models, and monitoring are the significant challenges facing IoT devices. This chapter addresses protection and confidentiality problems for IoT devices [57]. The authors of this document evaluated their proposed model's data security problems by referring to the five-dimensional model. The five-size data security model includes identity, requests, place, footage, and owner's privacy. It describes the summary of IoT devices and their context. This research also addressed IoT applications in various fields such as medical, smart homes, intelligent community protection framework, and IoT protocol stacks. The authors have clarified the protection and privacy of IoTs after discussing IoTs and their applications.

IoT security issues are sensors, front-end devices, networks, and IT back-end systems. Data security issues of IoTs include computer privacy, contact privacy, and processing privacy associated with addressing the IoT risks, IoT security threats, and many open problems in the IoT sector [58]. The information security and privacy of mobile medicines on IOS and Android were listed by Dehling et al. [59]. Different types of mHealth apps collect and supply vital, sensitive, private medical information that focuses primarily on the safety and privacy of mHealth apps. The findings indicate that 95.63% of applications are subject to such damages due to the protection of information and privacy concerns. Most data are stored in software in the cloud or storage application. Patient information protection and privacy in healthcare applications are significantly at risk [60], which focuses on wireless sensors networks in healthcare. The authors addressed how the sensors are obtained from patients and in the wireless network and addresses these applications' protection and privacy concerns. The authors pointed out the problems need to be made public, and government bodies, research institutes, and producers need to resolve such difficulties to enforce them. The standard WLAN architecture in healthcare applications in Figure 8.9 illustrates internet interactions with the wireless network. Wireless transfer of the data obtained by the sensors to the gateway and the portal then transmits the data directly to the server or the cloud network. It is always available to everyone via the internet.

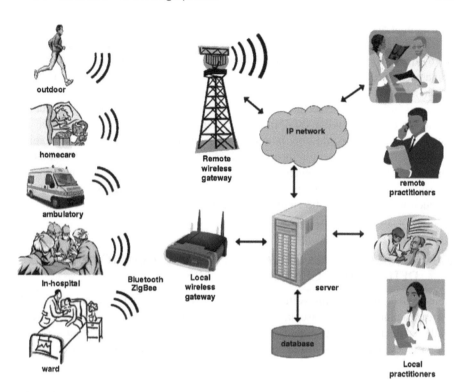

FIGURE 8.9   Typical architecture of wireless sensor networks in healthcare applications [60].

8.5   CHALLENGE OF IOT IN THE HEALTHCARE FIELD

IoMT devices have many integrated threats and obstacles, as well as advantages. The main research issues concern protection and privacy, lack of standards, limited interoperability, regulatory climate, and health concerns, i.e., lack of confidence, mal-administration, and technical debt, which is further clarified in various fields [61].

As IoMT is expected to be experiencing rapid growth over the next couple of years, an attractive goal for attackers would be the IoT healthcare domain. Safety risks will increase with IoT devices having a more feasible area for attack [12]. Lindman and Saarikko [9] emphasise IoT security threats that may remain unnoticed for relatively long periods, as IoTdevices function more independently or entirely independently from desktop computers and smartphones. Michalakis and Caridakis [62] state that the consumer's protection and privacy in the IoT solution in the healthcare sector are even more relevant. More IoMT devices are connected to global information networks; it is difficult to build highly scalable security systems without sacrificing security devices. As IoMT devices collect and produce vast quantities of data, the growing number of connected devices poses a risk of data protection breaches as the processing, mining, and provision of data over the internet is carried out. Yin et al. [10] called for more study in security and confidentiality management and complex trust.

Lindman and Saarikko [9] address the possible challenge to IoT due to the lack of standardisation of several different providers but not due to a transparent interface for communicating with various equipment. As a result, manufacturers create their contact protocols, which often provide little protection from unauthorised access. Farahani et al. [12] emphasise how a specialist community should concentrate on standardising healthcare technologies and consider a broad range of topics, such as layers for communication, equipment interfaces, interfaces to aggregate data, and gateway interfaces. In addition, failure to meet standards can lead to interoperability problems. Apart from requirements, the IoMT suppliers must consider regulations since several regulatory agencies control IoT. It was difficult to adopt new models focusing on the constant production of data, particularly in the face of a timeline from production to implementation and usage, because of the regulatory environment regulating conventional medical devices.

8.6   IOT SOLUTION FOR COVID-19 CRISIS: MONITORING AND DETECTION TECHNOLOGIES

Remote patient monitoring systems gather health data and vital information from the system, including cardiovascular rhythm, weight, blood pressure, and oxygen level. Gathered data is passed to clinicians to track patients remotely and intervene, if necessary. Remote patient monitoring can often be used in apps and medical wearables to monitor patients outside the conventional clinical setting by physicians and hospitals. Contactless or medical devices are available for remote control [15, 63].

8.6.1   CONTACTLESS MONITORING

The Binah.ai app is a healthcare apps with some unique elements. This video-based app removes the need for wearable and provides vital signs measurement such as heart rate, heart rate variability, mental stress, oxygen saturation, respiration rate, and all with medical-grade accuracy [64].

Binah.ai's service covers a wide range of fields, including telemedicine, remote patient care, primary treatment, preventive treatment, homes, and life insurance. Binah.ai provides a unique health research platform with its range of non-invasive, video-based health and wellness tracking solutions. Its technology turns any system with a simple camera into a physician-friendly tool. With this binah.ai app, patients remain in direct contact with the doctor. Patients can visit a doctor via video and this leads to a successful avoidance of the fatal Covid-19 viruses.

8.6.2   ABBOT ID NOW TECHNOLOGY

The fastest molecular care point check available for novel coronavirus (Covid-19) provides just five minutes of positive results and 13 minutes of negative result consequences. ID NOW is a reliable isothermal system based on instruments to detect infectious conditions in qualitative terms is called Abbot ID [65]. The innovative ID NOW platform delivers molecular results within minutes to make successful clinical decision-making faster.

8.6.3 BIOMEME

Scientists discovered a different way to minimise contact. The new BIOMEME app makes our smartphone a mobile laboratory for advanced diagnosis of DNA and real-time monitoring of diseases [66]. A docking plant for PCR (polymerase chain response) is included in the BIOMEME system. The mobile app monitors and analyses the system's performance. The mobile application provides specific test kits for sample preparation and detecting diseases or pathogens with their distinctive DNA or RNA signatures. The advanced platform complies with the gold standard that the most advanced central laboratories in the world use but does not need laboratory equipment or unique experience.

The inexpensive, user-facilitated program allows mobile testing for mobile clinics, disease tracking, and home use at the point of need for healthcare. Through mobile devices, Biomeme enables pharmaceutical companies to develop pop-up laboratories around the world conveniently. The mobile end-to-end platform of Biomeme enables users to carry PCRs wherever they need, from sample collection to data management. The SARS-CoV-2 tests allow RNA detection of the COVID-19-related severe acute respiratory syndrome 2. The RNA targets for coronaviruses have been multiplied by eliminating RNA and RT-PCR (MS2) by Biomeme [67]. Each order includes the exogenous positive controls, and all of them are immune (15–30C). Each reaction contains the following triplex lyophilised master mix, multiplexed primers, and probes:

- SARS-CoV-2-Orf1ab gene
- SARS-CoV-2-S gene
- RNA Process Control (RNA extraction and RT-PCR control utilising MS2 bacteriophage)

To date, the infection cannot be prevented or treated with a vaccine or antiviral drug. Furthermore, patients with Covid-19 infections are likely to be cross-infected by other patients and the medical team. Novel coronavirus-affected individuals have signs of fever, cough, and respiratory shortness. These people need ongoing health monitoring, particularly their body temperature, respiratory rate, and heart rate. Using a traditional method to track the patient's body temperature using an oral thermometer can increase viral transmission risk when these common infections are present.

8.6.4 VIVALNK

A leading provider of connected healthcare solutions for hospital and remote patient monitoring, VivaLNK, has developed a wearable sensor to track body temperature continuously. The sensor is easy to measure the temperature and monitor the temperature in real time. It is placed under the patient's arm. Information is sent from the patient to a centralised table of monitoring and assessing their medical personnel and physicians' lives. Recently, VivaLNK's continuous body temperature sensor has been used by the Shanghai Public Health Clinical Center (SPHCC) to fight the spread of coronavirus in China [68, 69].

VivaLNK has deliberately selected Cassia Networks [70] Bluetooth Gateways in conjunction with Yijin Health to offer a comprehensive health monitoring solution to SPHCC. For continuous body temperature surveillance, Bluetooth Cassias gateways relay the patient's vitality from a nurse's temperature sensor. This system not only eliminates the need for physical daily patient inspections but reduce the risk of cross-infection and also removes some of the medical personnel's burdens. Cassia Bluetooth gateways can cover two to six rooms, receiving data from up to 200 VivaLNK temperature sensors from one portal simultaneously.

8.6.5 SMART IMAGE READING SYSTEM TECHNOLOGY

The AI analysers system can carry out a comparative analysis of the different CT scans by the same patient, and changes in lesions can be measured [71]. It lets doctors track the disease's progression, assess the care, and have patient prognosis; mostly, it allows doctors to identify, triage quickly, and evaluate COVID-19 patients. Smart picture-reading technology enables remote AI reading by medical professionals outside of the epidemic.

8.6.6 PHONE APPS AND ELECTRONIC WRISTBAND

Governments worldwide use resources to identify where contagious individuals are and monitor quarantines. Countries and cities worldwide seek to promote "social distance" and reduce contact between individuals. The Singapore government launched a device known as TraceTogether, as shown in Figure [72]. Bluetooth signals between mobile phones are used to determine whether potential coronaviral carriers are in close contact with others. On March 20, 2020, the city-state launched an app that named it an additional resource to track communications based on infected people's alerts and memory. Contact tracking is the process by which people with close contact with infected patients are identified. In Hong Kong, citizens must wear a wristband linked to a smartphone app to alert officials if a person leaves quarantine. In its efforts to improve the quarantine and decrease the coronavirus spread, Hong Kong uses electronic bracelets.

8.6.7 MASIMO SAFETY NET

The Covid-19 pandemic has created a worldwide market for home-based surveillance and patient interaction solutions. Today the WHO recommends triage and monitoring Covid-19 patients based on temperature, breathing rate, and oxygen saturation by incorporating existing technology to provide a cloud-based solution; Masimo addresses this growing need [73]. The integrated solution of Masimo Safety Net provides continuous tether tracking, less pulse oximetry, and breathing rate together with a patient monitoring network, as shown in Figure 8.10. The Masimo Safety Net mobile application is securely sent via Bluetooth patient data. Reliable, Accurate Software Control System Reliable. To overcome traditional pulse oximetry by preserving precision in the presence of motion and low perfusions, Masimo has been equipped with advanced signal processing. Today, Masimo has been estimated to be used in leading hospitals and healthcare facilities around the world, with over

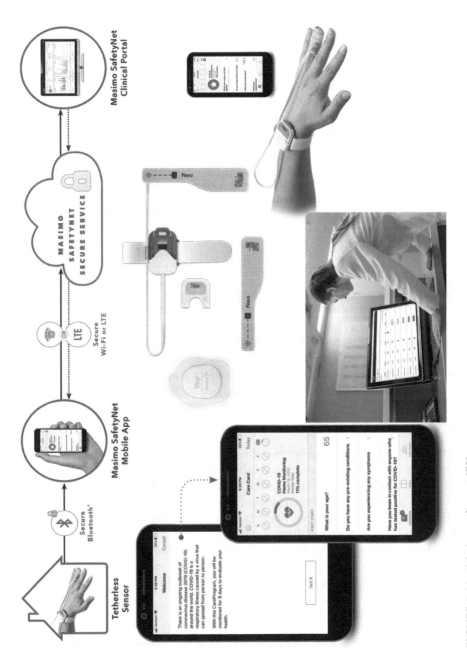

FIGURE 8.10 Masimo safety net [73].

200 million patients. The availability of a constant respiratory rate from the full range (RRp) and Masimo can also help clinicians monitor breathing rate without using an additional sensor.

8.6.8 COLOUR CODING (CHINA)

The Chinese government has joined hands with tech giants Alibaba and Tencent to develop a colour-coded health rating system that tracks millions of people every day, using its elaborate and expensive surveillance network for the public good. In collaboration with Alibaba, the smartphone app was first developed in Hangzhou. This classifies people based on their travel and medical history into three colours, white, yellow, or red. Similar software was developed by Tencent in the Shenzhen industrial centre [74]. The colour code is used to decide whether a person should be quarantined or accepted for public use. Only those with a green colour code can use the designated QR code in a public sphere such as offices, the metro, and other stations. The code and body temperature are regulated and used by more than 200 Chinese cities and spread nationwide at most public places.

8.6.9 BOSCH'S RAPID TEST

Patients usually need to wait for one to two days for an answer in studies currently being used. In the fight against Coronavirus, time is critical [75]. The Bosch quick test is one of the world's first fully automated molecular diagnostic tests that healthcare institutions can use directly. Within 2.5 hours from the time the sample is taken, the results to detect SARS-CoV-2 coronavirus infection are made available. This system may reduce the need to retain valuable time samples. It also ensures that patients easily gain trust in their health while quickly identifying and isolating infected individuals.

8.7 SUMMARY

In this chapter, we presented a summary of IoT resources and innovations in healthcare. Many research issues have been established, which are expected to become significant research trends in the coming years. A variety of research advantages have been identified, and the most important application fields are presented. We hope this study will enable researchers and practitioners to understand the tremendous potential of IoT in the medical field and detect significant challenges within IoMT. This work will also enable researchers to understand IoT applications in the healthcare sector to hinder and monitor the spreading of the Covid-19 virus and play an essential role in saving the world from this crisis pandemic.

REFERENCES

1. Zikria, Y.B., et al. *Internet of Things (IoT) operating systems management: opportunities, challenges, and solution*, 2019. Multidisciplinary Digital Publishing Institute.
2. Qadri, Y.A., et al. "The future of healthcare Internet of things: A survey of emerging technologies," *IEEE Communications Surveys & Tutorials*, 22(2), 2020, 1121–1167.

3. Aceto, G., Persico, V., Pescapé, A. "The role of information and communication technologies in healthcare: Taxonomies, perspectives, and challenges," *Journal of Network and Computer Applications*, 107, 2018, 125–154.

4. Dilsizian, S.E., Siegel, E.L. "Artificial intelligence in medicine and cardiac imaging: harnessing big data and advanced computing to provide personalised medical diagnosis and treatment," *Current Cardiology Reports*, 16(1), 2014, 441.

5. Hemingway, H. et al. "Big data from electronic health records for early and late translational cardiovascular research: challenges and potential," *European Heart Journal*, 39(16), 2018, 1481–1495.

6. Pearson, T. "How to replicate Watson hardware and systems design for your own use in your basement," 2011, www. ibm. com/developerworks/community/blogs. InsideSystemStorage/entry/ibm_watson_how_to_build_your_own_watson_jr_in_your_basement7.

7. Abdullah, A., et al., "Real time wireless health monitoring application using mobile devices," *International Journal of Computer Networks & Communications (IJCNC)*, 7(3), 2015, 13–30.

8. Lee, I., Lee, K. "The Internet of Things (IoT): Applications, investments, and challenges for enterprises," *Business Horizons*, 58(4), 2015, 431–440.

9. Lindman, J., Saarikko, T. "Towards an Internet of Things society: Perspectives from government agencies in Sweden," in *Proceedings of the 52nd Hawaii international conference on system sciences*, 2019.

10. Yuehong, Y., et al. "The Internet of things in healthcare: An overview," *Journal of Industrial Information Integration*, 1, 2016, 3–13.

11. Bouhaï, N., Saleh, I. "Internet of Things," *Iso-Britannia*, 2017. Wiley-ISTE.

12. Farahani, B., et al. "Towards fog-driven IoTeHealth: Promises and challenges of IoT in medicine and healthcare," *Future Generation Computer Systems*, 78, 2018, 659–676.

13. Porter, M.E., Heppelmann, J.E. "How smart, connected products are transforming competition," *Harvard Business Review*, 92(11), 2014, 64–88.

14. Al-Humairi, S.N.S., Kamal, A.A.A. "Design a smart infrastructure monitoring system: a response in the age of COVID-19 pandemic," *Innovative Infrastructure Solutions*, 6(3), 2021, 1–10.

15. Al-Humairi, S.N.S., Kamal, A.A.A. "Opportunities and challenges for the building monitoring systems in the age-pandemic of COVID-19: Review and prospects," *Innovative Infrastructure Solutions*, 6(2), 2021, 1–10.

16. Iyawa, G., Botha, A., Herselman, M. *Identifying and defining the terms and elements related to a digital health innovation ecosystem*, 2016. CSIR.

17. Lupton, D. "Health promotion in the digital era: a critical commentary," *Health promotion international*, 30(1), 2014, 174–183.

18. Meskó, B., et al. "Digital health is a cultural transformation of traditional healthcare," *Mhealth*, 3, 2017.

19. Kulkarni, A., Sathe, S. "Healthcare applications of the Internet of Things: A review," *International Journal of Computer Science and Information Technologies*, 5(5), 2014, 6229–6232.

20. Laplante, P.A., Laplante, N. "The Internet of Things in healthcare: Potential applications and challenges," *It Professional*, 18(3), 2016, 2–4.

21. Chang, C.K., Oyama, K. "Guest editorial: a roadmap for mobile and cloud services for digital health," *IEEE Transactions on Services Computing*, 11(2), 2018, 232–235.

22. Basatneh, R., Najafi, B., Armstrong, D.G. "Health sensors, smart home devices, and the Internet of medical things: an opportunity for dramatic improvement in care for

the lower extremity complications of diabetes," *Journal of Diabetes Science and Technology*, 12(3), 2018, 577–586.

23. Hassanalieragh, M., et al. "Health monitoring and management using Internet-of-Things (IoT) sensing with cloud-based processing: Opportunities and challenges," in *2015 IEEE International Conference on Services Computing*, 2015. IEEE.

24. Dimitrov, D.V. "Medical internet of things and big data in healthcare," *Healthcare Informatics Research*, 22(3), 2016, 156–163.

25. Albahri, O., et al. "Systematic review of real-time remote health monitoring system in triage and priority-based sensor technology: Taxonomy, open challenges, motivation and recommendations," *Journal of Medical Systems*, 42(5), 2018, 80.

26. Jagadeeswari, V., et al. "A study on medical Internet of Things and Big Data in personalised healthcare system," *Health Information Science and Systems*, 6(1), 2018, 14.

27. Sun, W., et al. "Security and privacy in the medical Internet of things: A review," *Security and Communication Networks*, 2018.

28. Irfan, M., Ahmad, N. "Internet of medical things: Architectural model, motivational factors and impediments," in *2018 15th Learning and Technology Conference (L&T)*, 2018. IEEE.

29. Rao, M., et al. "Future challenges, benefits of Internet of medical things and applications in healthcare domain," *Journal of Communications*, 12(4), 2020.

30. Sawand, A., et al. "Toward energy-efficient and trustworthy eHealth monitoring system," *China Communications*, 12(1), 2015, 46–65.

31. Puustjarvi, J., Puustjarvi, L. "Personal health ontology: Towards the interoperation of e-health tools," *International Journal of Electronic Healthcare*, 6(1), 2011, 62–75.

32. Puustjärvi, J., Puustjärvi, L. "Automating remote monitoring and information therapy: An opportunity to practice telemedicine in developing countries," in *2011 IST-Africa Conference Proceedings*, 2011. IEEE.

33. Alahmadi, A., Soh, B. "A smart approach towards a mobile e-health monitoring system architecture," in *2011 International Conference on Research and Innovation in Information Systems*, 2011. IEEE.

34. Archer, N., Cocosila, M. "A comparison of physician pre-adoption and adoption views on electronic health records in Canadian medical practices," *Journal of Medical Internet Research*, 13(3), 2011, e57.

35. Mukherjee, S., Dolui, K., Datta, S.K. "Patient health management system using e-health monitoring architecture," in *2014 IEEE international advance computing conference (IACC)*, 2014. IEEE.

36. Szakacs-Simon, P., Moraru, S., Perniu, L. "Android application developed to extend health monitoring device range and real-time patient tracking," in *2013 IEEE 9th international conference on computational cybernetics (ICCC)*, 2013. IEEE.

37. Ha, M., Lim, S., Ko, H. "Wearable and flexible sensors for user-interactive health-monitoring devices," *Journal of Materials Chemistry B*, 6(24), 2018, 4043–4064.

38. Butca, C.G., et al. "Wearable sensors and cloud platform for monitoring environmental parameters in e-health applications," in *2014 11th international symposium on electronics and telecommunications (ISETC)*, 2014. IEEE.

39. Suryani, V., et al. "Electrocardiagram monitoring on OpenMTC platform," in *38th annual IEEE conference on local computer networks-workshops*, 2013. IEEE.

40. Fletcher, R.R., et al. "iCalm: Wearable sensor and network architecture for wirelessly communicating and logging autonomic activity," *IEEE Transactions on Information Technology in Biomedicine*, 14(2), 2010, 215–223.

41. Luxner, A.J., *A mobile device-controlled blood pressure monitor*, 2013. San Diego State University.
42. Agrawal, A., *Initial validation of withings pulse wave velocity and body composition scale*, 2017. Appalachian State University.
43. Miranda, D., Calderón, M., Favela, J. "Anxiety detection using wearable monitoring," in *Proceedings of the 5th Mexican conference on human-computer interaction*, 2014.
44. Pizzo, A.D., et al. "Sport experience design: Wearable fitness technology in the health and fitness industry," *Journal of Sport Management*, 1(aop), 2020, 1–14.
45. Di Serio, A., et al. "Potential of sub-GHz wireless for future IoTwearables and design of compact 915 MHz antenna," *Sensors*, 18(1), 2018, 22.
46. Hello. "Helo Wristband gives the peace of mind that everyone is healthy and safe by monitoring the information," 2020, https://helolifestyle.net.
47. Monitor. "WBP Healthcare wearable market which could help you live a healthier and better life, when it comes to health wearables it tracks the real-time information, 2020, http://medicalfuturist.com/top-healthcare-wearables/.
48. Halcox, J.P., et al. "Assessment of remote heart rhythm sampling using the AliveCor heart monitor to screen for atrial fibrillation: the REHEARSE-AF study," *Circulation*, 136(19), 2017, 1784–1794.
49. Kakria, P., Tripathi, N., Kitipawang, P. "A real-time health monitoring system for remote cardiac patients using smartphone and wearable sensors," *International Journal of Telemedicine and Applications*, 2015.
50. Vukotic, A., Goodwill, J., *Apache Tomcat 7*, 2011: Springer.
51. Dehling, T., Sunyaev, A. "Architecture and design of a patient-friendly eHealth web application: patient information leaflets and supplementary services," in *Proceedings of the 18th Americas conference on information systems (AMCIS 2012)*, 2012.
52. Weider, D.Y., et al. "A security oriented design (SOD) framework for ehealth systems," in *2014 IEEE 38th international computer software and applications conference workshops*, 2014. IEEE.
53. Winesett, J., *Web Application development with Yii and PHP*, 2012. Packt Publishing Ltd.
54. Hogan, M., et al. "Nist cloud computing standards roadmap," *NIST Special Publication*, 35, 2011, 6–11.
55. Wang, J., et al. "Smartphone interventions for long-term health management of chronic diseases: an integrative review," *Telemedicine and e-Health*, 20(6), 2014, 570–583.
56. Mishra, S.M., *Wearable android: Android wear and Google fit app development*, 2015. John Wiley & Sons.
57. Ankitha, S., Balajee, M. "Security and Privacy Issues in IoT," *SCIREA Journal of Agriculture*, 1(2), 2016, 135–142.
58. Abomhara, M., Køien, G.M. "Security and privacy in the Internet of Things: Current status and open issues," in *2014 international conference on privacy and security in mobile systems (PRISMS)*, 2014. IEEE.
59. Dehling, T., et al. "Exploring the far side of mobile health: information security and privacy of mobile health apps on iOS and Android," *JMIR mHealth and uHealth*, 3(1), 2015, e8.
60. Al Ameen, M., Liu, J., Kwak, K. "Security and privacy issues in wireless sensor networks for healthcare applications," *Journal of Medical Systems*, 36(1), 2012, 93–101.
61. Al-Humairi, S., et al., *COVID-19 PANDEMIC: Monitoring technologies. healthcare and panic buying behaviour*, 2020. White Falcon Publishing.

62. Michalakis, K., Caridakis, G. " IoT Contextual Factors on Healthcare," *Journal of Advances in Experimental Medicine and Biology*, 2017, 989, 189–200.

63. Al-Humairi, S.N.S., et al. "Conceptual design: A novel Covid-19 smart AI helmet," *Int J EmergTechnol*, 11(5), 2020, 389–396.

64. Desk, A.N. "Binah.ai Delivers AI-Powered, Non-Contact," *Video-Based Health and Wellness Monitoring Solutions*, 2019; www.aithority.com/technology/big-data/binah-ai-delivers-ai-powered-non-contact-video-based-health-and-wellness-monitoring-solutions/.

65. Park, A. "Abbott launches molecular point-of-care test to detect novel coronavirus in as little as five minutes," 2020, https://abbott.mediaroom.com/2020-03-27-Abbott-Launc hes-Molecular-Point-of-Care-Test-to-Detect-Novel-Coronavirus-in-as-Little-as-Five-Minutes.

66. DeJohn, M.D., Wilson, J. vanWestrienen, Maksutovic, M., *Analytic device*, 2020, Google Patents.

67. Nicolematthesen. "Coronavirus Test Available Now as COVID-19 Spreads Worldwide," 2020, www.sep.benfranklin.org/2020/03/13/coronavirus-test-available-now-as-covid-19-spreads-worldwide/.

68. Campbell, C., "VivaLNK Offers Rapid Deployment Remote Patient Monitoring Solution with Alibaba," 2020, www.prnewswire.com/news-releases/vivalnk-offers-rapid-deployment-remote-patient-monitoring-solution-with-alibaba-301013155.html.

69. Pennic, F. "Shanghai Public Health Clinical Center Uses Wearable Sensors to Combat Spread of Coronavirus in China," 2020, https://hitconsultant.net/2020/01/31/shanghai-public-health-clinical-wearable-sensors-coronavirus-in-china/#.XpvStS-w3Nw.

70. Gao, F., et al., *Methods, devices, and systems for supporting wireless roaming*, 2019, Google Patents.

71. Bernheim, A., et al. "Chest CT findings in coronavirus disease-19 (COVID-19): Relationship to duration of infection," *Radiology*, 2020, 200463.

72. Cho, H., Ippolito, D., Yu, Y.W. "Contact tracing mobile apps for covid-19: Privacy considerations and related trade-offs," *arXiv preprint arXiv*:2003.11511, 2020.

73. Costello, J., et al., *Massena Memorial Hospital of New York adopts Masimo Root® and Masimo Patient SafetyNet™*, 2020. EMR.

74. Lin, L. "China Turns to Health-Rating Apps to Control Movements During Coronavirus Outbreak," 2020, www.wsj.com/articles/china-turns-to-health-rating-apps-to-control-movements-during-coronavirus-outbreak-11582046508.

75. Solutions, B.H. "Vivalytic VRI Test," 2020, www.bosch-healthcare.com/en/whats-new/news/vivalytic-test-for-covid-19/.

9 How Artificial Intelligence and IoT Are Facing Covid-19
An Overview

Wahida Handouzi
LAT Laboratory
Tlemcen University

Kaouter Karboub
FRDISI and ENSEM
Hassan II University

Mohamed Tabaa
LPRI EMSI Casablanca

CONTENTS

The end of 2019 was marked by the appearance of the new coronavirus (Covid-19) in Wuhan-China. The new virus was declared a pandemic in March 2020 by the World Health Organization (WHO). Now, this has forced countries worldwide to limit daily living activities by imposing a lockdown. This situation has prompted the scientific community to focus on the emergence of artificial intelligence, deep learning, and IoT to offer solutions that facilitate daily life in front of the challenges

DOI: 10.1201/9781003146087-12

imposed by sanitary confinement. The medical field emitted strong demand because of the shortage of screening tests for diagnostic systems via multimodal databases. Also, digital tracing systems, real-time propagation monitoring systems, etc. This chapter presents an overview of these systems, applications, and all the important contributions in this area and emphasizes their incidence in the fight against Covid-19 propagation. Also, we will propose directions and identify challenges that can help improve the management of such crises.

9.1   INTRODUCTION

What is coronavirus? It is an illness that mostly causes fever, dry cough, fatigue etc. [1]. This disease is related to the newly discovered strain of SARS. People with pre-existing medical conditions (cardiovascular disease, diabetes, chronic respiratory disease, and cancer) and older people are the most likely to develop a severe illness due to the virus [1] [2].

The virus was declared a pandemic on March 11, 2020, by the WHO after more than 100 countries declared having more than 118,000 cases of the disease and over 4,200 deaths [3]. This health crisis caused an unprecedented socio-economic crisis leaving longstanding and deep scars worldwide. It has turn upside down the countries that it touches, especially Third World countries [4], [5], [6]. The volume of China merchandise trade was down 17% in the first two months of 2020 [7]. Not forgetting that the same impact on international relations may also push firms to retreat from globalization and replace it with shortened supply chains and suppliers located in the same country to avoid any further disruption in their activity [8]. As a result, governments of many countries have proposed a set of interventions that may limit Covid-19 consequences.

The collaboration of New Approaches to Economic Challenges (NAEC group) with Organisation for Economic Cooperation and Development (OECD) has led to a report that defines concepts related to systematic threats and reviews the analytical and governance strategies to face these threats [9]. Despite experience with other pandemics (black plague, Spanish flu of 1918, HIV and influenza A (H1N1) of 2009), the world has been caught off guard by this new virus. Social distancing policies have had to be introduced because knowledge about its behaviour and the best ways to manage it was inadequate.

In less than a year, 53,853,718 cases of Covid-19 have been reported following the standard definition of a case and testing strategies applied in affected countries. This includes 1,293,106 deaths and 37,593,422 recovered Covid-19 patients globally [10]. However, the actual number of infections may be higher since the capacity of some countries to do reliable screening tests is low. To know how Covid-19 is spreading, we have to know the counts of confirmed cases and how much a country tests. We cannot understand the pandemic without this information and know which countries are reacting well to combating it [11]. Public health responses against Covid-19 have included strong testing capacity, quick isolation of positive cases, effective contact tracing, and quarantine of identified contacts; also, social distancing and compulsory wearing a mask for all individuals in public places.

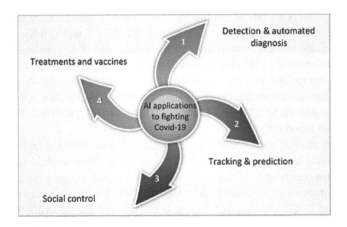

FIGURE 9.1 Some applications of AI for fighting Covid-19.

The screening test validated by the WHO is the polymerase chain reaction test (PCR) [12], which may or may not show RNA (ribonucleic acid = assembly of ribonucleotides) viral in a nasopharyngeal swab obtained. This test makes it possible to specify whether, at an instant (T), the person is a carrier of the virus or not. The results are obtained in a few hours, or even more quickly following the development of devices making it possible to obtain a result in less than an hour. This test is performed and analysed by a specialist to confirm the diagnosis [8].

More than ever, there is a huge need for new technologies like artificial intelligence (AI) to support public health and help deal with this critical situation and help minimize the burden on specialized laboratories, medical staff, and somehow reduce the impact of the economic crisis. From all of this, artificial intelligence emerges in several directions (Figure 9.1) to facing this situation, detection and automated diagnosis, tracking and prediction, social control and treatments and vaccines.

9.2   EXISTING CONTRIBUTIONS OF AI AGAINST COVID-19

This section aims to review how AI can present a potential tool for decision-making to analyse and prepare for prevention and response against the virus. We explore different databases to find publications with a focus on evidence-based research articles.

9.2.1   AI FOR AUTOMATIC DETECTION OF COVID-19

The limited number of Covid-19 test kits in hospitals due to increased demand and the urge to test more cases daily made it critical to develop an automatic detection system as a rapid means of identifying cases. AI can detect, diagnose and prevent the spread of the virus. How? Through algorithms capable of identifying potential features and anomalies such as recognition systems and computer vision. A paper published in March 2020 [13] presents a CNN-based approach to identify Covid-19 cases. The proposed solution is a CNN algorithm and AlexNet as a transfer deep learning algorithm [14]. The first extracts relevant features from 361 CT and 170 X-ray images.

In contrast, the second aims to transfer the knowledge of the pre-trained AlexNet model to this specific case with modification. Used input images are resized and unified according to the Alex Net model to fit the 227-227-3 as width-height-channel, while parameters of the modified network are configured as follows: batch size to 10, the number of epochs to 20, learning rate initialized to 3e-4, shuffling is set at every epoch and validation frequency to 3.

As in such studies used images, other works included blood samples as in [15]. This study used blood samples from 375 confirmed cases to develop the model consisting of a supervised XGBoost classifier. The blood samples used in the study were first split into a 70% training and a 30% test set, then cross-validated five times. The data used in the training and testing uses only the last recordings taken from patients during their stay in the hospital. As claimed by the authors, such a procedure gives the model more visibility on parameters associated with the study. The model highlighted lactic dehydrogenase (LDH), lymphocyte and high-sensitivity C-reactive protein (hs-CRP) as three important factors that might predict the survival of individuals with an accuracy of 90% that shows that the model can be applied to any blood sample. The authors also confirmed the results as "far" from a patient clinical outcome. Furthermore, as the proposed machine learning method is a data-driven study, the authors mentioned that changes in the data (size or nature) might engender changes in the model outcomes.

In [16], authors suggested that artificial intelligence algorithms can support the increasing diagnosis demand and lack of resources. Such support can be achieved by combining chest-computed tomography findings with clinical symptoms, exposure history, and laboratory testing. The authors also proposed a joint AI algorithm combining CT images and clinical history. They achieved 0.92 of AUC and 84.3% sensitivity compared to a senior thoracic radiologist, 74.6%. The authors applied the approach to a test set of 279 cases, and 90 out of 134 were correctly classified.

While [17] conducted research aiming to build a deep learning system to detect Covid-19 pneumonia on high resolution computed tomography. The deep learning model showed comparable performance with expert radiologists. Such a study included 46,096 anonymous CT scan images from 106 admitted patients. The model, namely UNet ++, was first trained to extract features from images then, on detecting suspicious areas, which resulted in classifying infected and uninfected patients.

In this study, three different models based on convolutional neural networks (ResNet50, InceptionV3 and InceptionResNetV2) were proposed to detect Covid-19-infected patients using chest x-rays [18]. The preformed models have shown very high results in the small data set (50 Covid-19 vs 50 Normal). Especially, the performed ResNet50 model achieved the highest accuracy with 98% compared with the two other models.

The authors of this study have developed and tested a novel computer-assisted diagnosis (CAD) system. The study includes several images preprocessing algorithms to remove diaphragms, normalize the image contrast or noise ratio, and generate three images as inputs. The images are then inputted to a convolutional neural network

TABLE 9.1
Summary of Some Studies Investigated the Early Detection of Covid-19

Authors	Dataset	Used Model	Results
[20]	RSNA pneumonia dataset [21] chest X-Ray [22]	Transfer learning ResNet-101 ResNet-152	96.1%
[19]	Covid-19, normal (from healthy persons), viral pneumonia and bacterial pneumonia	ResNet50, ResNet101, ResNet152, InceptionV3 and Inception-ResNetV2	ResNet50 gave the best performance with an accuracy, recall and specificity of 98%, 96%, and 100% respectively
[23]	Evaluate the performance of convolutional neural network architectures	Transfer learning	the best precision, sensitivity and specificity obtained are respectively 96.78%, 98.66% and 96.46%
[24]	Building a Computer Assisted Diagnostic (CAD) web service to detect COVID19 online	(DenseNet121 InceptionV3 ResNet50V2 ResNet50V1 MobileNetV1 MobileNetV2)	The best DenseNet121 architecture which gave 90.80% recall rate, 89.76% accuracy and 90.61% accuracy.
[25]	Multiple international thoracic CT datasets	2D and 3D deep learning models	0.996 AUC (95%CI: 0.989-1.00)

based on transfer learning (a CNN network based on VGG16) to classify them into three classes of pneumonia infected with Covid-19 [19].

Other studies that investigate the early detection of Covid-19 using deep learning architectures are shown in Table 9.1.

9.2.2 TRACKING AND PREDICTION

Covid-19 is just another illustration of how systems are connected and can change each other. A range of social, economic, and environmental changes and, more specifically, practices cause a whole change in the natural order of things. Such change is the same that caused a virus to be able to transmit from animals to humans. Covid-19 has had tremendous effects on the health systems, economies and social balance of the world since the first detected case in Wuhan, China, in December 2019.

According to its latest reports, the WHO declared that the virus had infected more than 28 million people all around the globe, more than 70% of them recovered. In contrast, more than 3.25% of them died, and 7,087,234 are active cases, of which 99% are considered a mild condition, and 1% are severe or critical [26]. The balance sheets are rising inexorably as European countries increase restrictions to stem the

TABLE 9.2
World Region Situation in Numbers to November 14, 2020 [10]

	Global Cases	Global Deaths	Global Recovery	Critical Cases
Africa	1,961,168	46,907	1,650,880	2,540
Asia	14,937,913	264,036	13,320,284	24,367
South America	10,272,525	308,102	9,264,701	17,451
North America	13,075,552	374,252	8,298,545	36,188
Europe	13,563,740	317,218	5,025,462	29,062
Oceania	42,099	994	32,891	26
World	53,853,718	1,311,524	37,593,422	109,638

second wave of the epidemic. About a year after the beginning of the pandemic, approximately in November 2020, Spain crossed the threshold of 42,619 deaths on November 21, and the United Kingdom has 54,381 deaths. For its part, Italy has exceeded one million cases since the start of the epidemic, with 48,569 deaths [10] [27]. More details about cases per continent are shown in the following Table 9.2. We can see that many cases are registered in North America, especially in the United States, which is due to the number of realized tests, 177,231,071 [10].

All this data flow has made it possible to create dozens of dashboards giving the real-time situation of the spread of the pandemic using data visualization [27]–[30].

9.3 AI FOR SOCIAL CONTROL

Such policies demonstrate a significant need for science and technology. Many companies launched several challenges and developed specialized intelligent robots, drones, and wearables devices to support, improve and help ensure the functioning of the healthcare system among others. However, this is not only in the short term but can be considered long-term solutions. These robots are used to deliver food and medicine and to disinfect places. While smartphone applications also play an important part, not to replace human-to-human communication, but to manage, facilitate this communication, and keep people safe from any evitable contact [31] [32].

As the virus spreads rapidly and uncontrollably and its consequences start to choke countries possibility to fight over a long period, seeking new durable, supportive, trusted ways becomes very important. Artificial intelligence in the presence of big data and sensors feeding these databases can present a very promotive solution. It is important to mention that since the appearance of Covid-19, researchers oriented their research scope on different aspects and domains that might be affected by the pandemic. Doctors, radiologists, and healthcare professionals started gathering data by studying patients common symptoms, historical data, and other patterns.

On the other hand, scientists in the last few months also focused their interests on the possibility of using AI and AI-enabled robots to fight the new virus. To help overcome the limitations of the epidemiological model approach and help policymakers draw up a response plan, authors in [33] developed an AI-based method to forecast new and cumulative cases of Covid-19. The model gave high accuracy. While in [34], researchers used the NLP technique to analyse and extract related news features, such as epidemic control measures and citizens awareness about epidemic prevention. These features are the input of an LSTM model to update the infection rate calculated by the ISI model. Such a technique enables researchers and scientists to surpass epidemic models limitations due to single-factor data. The study uses the retrospective method to analyse the time laws of epidemic transmission in the past few days.

The hybrid artificial intelligence model suggested in this chapter for forecasting Covid-19 is integrated with the NLP module. In preventing a second epidemic wave in Guangdong and Zhejiang, the continued strategy of "early warning" and subsequent isolation may be successful. On February 10, 2020, the confirmed Covid-19 cases in Hubei, Guangdong, and Zhejiang provinces were 31,728, 1,177 and 1,117 respectively. In the case of a delay of five days in executing the measures, the initial rise in the proportion of exposed cases would have resulted in an exponential increase in infected cases [35].

An unprecedented rise in infection from novel coronavirus (Covid-19) marked the end of 2019 and the beginning of 2020. Telerobots, robotic vehicles with a human operator–remote control interface, provide the most noticeable advantage in terms of assistance to the healthcare sector. Facilitating the monitoring of patients as healthcare staff stays in a safe area, telehealth technology may minimize the time of interaction between patients and frontline healthcare workers [31], [36], [37]. Another example of the future application of robotic and autonomous devices is outsourcing labour-intensive manual processes [38], [39], [40], [41].

9.3.1 AI Helps to Develop Treatments and Vaccines against Covid-19

If you know the enemy and know yourself, you need not fear the result of a hundred battles. If you know yourself but not the enemy, you will also suffer a defeat for every victory gained. If you know neither the enemy nor yourself, you will succumb in every battle.

Sun Tz, *The Art of War*

This quote reflects perfectly the reality of Covid-19. Researchers from all over the globe found themselves confronted with the need to conduct several types of research and studies into this newly appearing infectious disease. Artificial intelligence can be of essential use in this case.

In [42], Wu et al.'s analysis using a whole genome collected from a patient who served at a seafood market in Wuhan City, Hubei Province, China, reveals that the virus is closely linked to a group of SARS-like CoVs. The findings of a phylogenetic analysis indicate that the virus belongs to the genus Beta coronavirus, subgenus Sarbecovirus.

Zhou et al. advocate for the possible bat origin of SARS-CoV-2 by using whole-genome sequences of five patients at the onset of the outbreak in Wuhan, China. Although in [43], this paper recorded all point mutations of SARS-CoV-2 after the first genomes of the virus were generated in December 2019. Among 3,089 D614G mutations, the prediction findings indicate that none of these mutations is likely to alter the secondary protein structure and the relative abundance of solvents. The SARS-CoV-2 mutation database is based on many genome sequences (6,324) from 45 countries. The authors predicted the secondary structure and relative solvent usability of the virus proteins to determine whether the mutations observed could alter the characteristics of the virus. These regions may be aimed for the production of vaccines and medicines.

Other experiments [44] have shown that it is possible to conclude which amino acid residues are in contact by covariation in homologous sequences, allowing predicting protein structures. The study shows that a neural network can be programmed to predict distances between pairs of residues that convey more structure information than touch predictions.

A study about protein structure prediction has shown that a simple gradient descent algorithm can produce structures without complicated sampling procedures. Four small molecule drugs were classified as recurring candidates against 2019-nCoV 24. They were selected through high-throughput statistical screening of 8,000 experimental and accepted drugs and small molecules in the library [45].

As the virus continues to spread and destroy the lives of thousands of people worldwide, the battle for a cure is continuing. In [46], authors have developed two deep learning models focused on low-dimensional algebraic topology representations of macromolecular complexes. The high structural similarity between the two proteases indicates that anti-SARS-CoV chemicals may be effective. According to the expected binding affinities, the authors proposed several FDA-approved drugs as potentially highly potent drugs.

Another line of research was undertaken by [47] that proposes using the benevolentAI knowledge graph, a large repository of medical structures based on machine learning to extract numerous connections from the literature. This underwent customizations for Covid-19. All of this is to identify approved drugs that can help block viral infection.

9.4   CONCLUSION AND FUTURE PROSPECTS

This chapter reviewed the contributions published in 2020 to deal with Covid-19 and using artificial intelligence technology. We focused on four areas where we believe that AI can make a big step forward in the fight against this pandemic and serve as a starting point to face other health crises.

We started with state of the art regarding the automatic detection of Covid via multimodal databases. We have noticed that many researchers have focused on this axis, given the importance of early detection of this pandemic.

Next, we hovered over existing real-time trackers using big data analysis and visualizations. These trackers allow us to know if anything has happened with the spread of the virus and to know when to reach the peak of contamination. Also, they help us see the impact of the containment put into effect by different countries and detect the best responses and measures to limit its spread.

We also have to analyse the contributions of artificial intelligence to maintaining social distance, which means using robots to approach cases with a positive diagnosis that will help limit contamination and protect public health workers. Their use remains minimal and could be better invested.

Finally, the use of artificial intelligence technology to design drugs and better understand the virus was analysed. This axis remains a field not very much used by experts who could push scientists to collaborate to enrich it with new techniques to revolutionize this field and make the response time faster.

Shortly before the end of 2020, we were facing the second wave of contamination globally due to the relaxation and failure to respect preventive measures several countries have decided to impose containment to curb the spread of Covid-19. To do this, knowledge of the existing contributions made available worldwide for the rapid and low-cost detection of the virus, the tracking of affected people and contaminations could help defeat Covid.

Finally, it took a health crisis to show the need to integrate artificial intelligence technologies into different areas of daily life. It would require reviewing the obstacles that we have identified, including insufficient data, the presence of ethical traps and the presence of legal obstacles.

REFERENCES

1. "Coronavirus disease (Covid-19)," www.who.int/news-room/q-a-detail/coronavirus-disease-covid-19 (accessed November 13, 2020).
2. CDC. "Coronavirus Disease 2019 (Covid-19) – Symptoms," *Centers for Disease Control and Prevention*, May 13, 2020. www.cdc.gov/coronavirus/2019-ncov/symptoms-testing/symptoms.html (accessed November 15, 2020).
3. "Coronavirus Disease (Covid-19) – events as they happen," 2000, www.who.int/emergencies/diseases/novel-coronavirus-2019/events-as-they-happen (accessed November 18, 2020).
4. Kofman, Y.B., Garfin D.R. "Home is not always a haven: The domestic violence crisis amid the Covid-19 pandemic," *Psychol. Trauma Theory Res. Pract. Policy*, 12(S1), 2020, S199, 20200601, doi: 10.1037/tra0000866.
5. Ozili, P.K. "Covid-19 Pandemic and Economic Crisis: The Nigerian Experience and Structural Causes," Social Science Research Network, Rochester, NY, SSRN Scholarly Paper ID 3567419, Apr. 2020. doi: 10.2139/ssrn.3567419.
6. ILO. "As jobs crisis deepens, ILO warns of uncertain and incomplete labour market recovery," 2020, www.ilo.org/global/about-the-ilo/newsroom/news/WCMS_749398/lang--en/index.htm (accessed November 14, 2020).
7. WEO. "World Economic Outlook (October 2020) – Real GDP growth," 2020, www.imf.org/external/datamapper/NGDP_RPCH@WEO (accessed November 21, 2020).
8. Jüttner, U., Maklan, S. "Supply chain resilience in the global financial crisis: an empirical study," *Supply Chain Manag. Int. J.*, 16(4), 2011, pp. 246–259, doi: 10.1108/13598541111139062.
9. Massaro, E., Ganin, A., Perra, N., Linkov, I., Vespignani, A. "Resilience management during large-scale epidemic outbreaks," *Sci. Rep.*, 8(1), 2018, 1859, doi: 10.1038/s41598-018-19706-2.
10. "Coronavirus Update (Live): 53,853,718 Cases and 1,311,524 Deaths from Covid-19 Virus Pandemic – Worldometer", 2020, www.worldometers.info/coronavirus/?utm_campaign=homeAdvegas1?#countries (accessed Nov. 14, 2020).

11. "Coronavirus (Covid-19) Testing – Statistics and Research," *Our World in Data*, 2020, https://ourworldindata.org/coronavirus-testing (accessed November 19, 2020).

12. Drosten, C. et al. "Identification of a novel coronavirus in patients with severe acute respiratory syndrome," *N. Engl. J. Med.*, 348(20), May 2003, 1967–1976, doi: 10.1056/NEJMoa030747.

13. Maghdid, H.S., Asaad, A.T., Ghafoor, K.Z., Sadiq, A.S., Khan, M.K. "Diagnosing Covid-19 pneumonia from X-Ray and CT images using deep learning and transfer learning algorithms," *ArXiv200400038 Cs Eess*, 2020, http://arxiv.org/abs/2004.00038 (accessed: November 21, 2020).

14. Krizhevsky, A., Sutskever, I., Hinton, G.E. "ImageNet classification with deep convolutional neural networks," *Commun. ACM*, 60(6), May 2017, 84–90, doi: 10.1145/3065386.

15. Yan, L. et al. "Prediction of survival for severe Covid-19 patients with three clinical features: development of a machine learning-based prognostic model with clinical data in Wuhan," *medRxiv*, Mar. 2020, p. 2020.02.27.20028027, doi: 10.1101/2020.02.27.20028027.

16. Mei, X. et al. "Artificial intelligence–enabled rapid diagnosis of patients with Covid-19," *Nat. Med.*, 26(8), art. no. 8, 2020, doi: 10.1038/s41591-020-0931-3.

17. Chen, J. et al. "Deep learning-based model for detecting 2019 novel coronavirus pneumonia on high-resolution computed tomography: a prospective study," *medRxiv*, Mar. 2020, 2020.02.25.20021568, doi: 10.1101/2020.02.25.20021568.

18. Narin, A., Kaya, C., Pamuk, Z. "Automatic Detection of Coronavirus Disease (Covid-19) Using X-ray Images and Deep Convolutional Neural Networks," *ArXiv200310849 Cs Eess*, 2020, http://arxiv.org/abs/2003.10849 (accessed: October 9, 2020).

19. Heidari, M., Mirniaharikandehei, S., Khuzani, A.Z., Danala, G., Qiu, Y., Zheng, B. "Improving performance of CNN to predict likelihood of Covid-19 using chest X-ray images with preprocessing algorithms," *Int. J. Med. Inf.*, 144, Dec. 2020, 104284, doi: 10.1016/j.ijmedinf.2020.104284.

20. Wang, N., Liu, H., Xu, C. "Deep Learning for The Detection of Covid-19 Using Transfer Learning and Model Integration," in *2020 IEEE 10th International Conference on Electronics Information and Emergency Communication (ICEIEC)*, Jul. 2020, pp. 281–284. doi: 10.1109/ICEIEC49280.2020.9152329.

21. "RSNA Pneumonia Detection Challenge," https://kaggle.com/c/rsna-pneumonia-detection-challenge (accessed October 9, 2020).

22. Cohen, J.P. *ieee8023/covid-chestxray-dataset*, 2020, https://github.com/ieee8023/covid-chestxray-dataset

23. Apostolopoulos, I.D., Bessiana, T. "Covid-19: Automatic detection from X-Ray images utilizing transfer learning with convolutional neural networks," *Phys. Eng. Sci. Med.*, 43(2), 2020, 635–640, doi: 10.1007/s13246-020-00865-4.

24. Saeedi, A., Saeedi, M., Maghsoudi, A. "A novel and reliable deep learning web-based tool to detect Covid-19 infection from chest CT-scan," *ArXiv200614419 Cs Eess*, Jun. 2020, http://arxiv.org/abs/2006.14419 (accessed: October 09, 2020)

25. Gozes, O. et al. "Rapid AI development cycle for the Coronavirus (Covid-19) pandemic: Initial results for automated detection & patient monitoring using deep learning CT image analysis," *ArXiv200305037 Cs Eess*, Mar. 2020, http://arxiv.org/abs/2003.05037.

26. WHO. "Coronavirus Disease (Covid-19) Situation Reports," www.who.int/emergencies/diseases/novel-coronavirus-2019/situation-reports (accessed November 21, 2020).

27. Dong, E., Du, H., Gardner, L. "An interactive web-based dashboard to track Covid-19 in real time," *Lancet Infect. Dis.*, 20(5), 2020, 533–534, doi: 10.1016/S1473-3099(20)30120-1.

28. Hadfield, J. et al. "Nextstrain: Real-time tracking of pathogen evolution," *Bioinformatics*, 34(23), 2018, pp. 4121–4123, doi: 10.1093/bioinformatics/bty407.

29. "HealthMap | Flu Map | Contagious Disease Surveillance | Virus Awareness." http://healthmap.org (accessed November 21, 2020).

30. Sagulenko, P., Puller, V., Neher, R.A. "TreeTime: Maximum-likelihood phylodynamic analysis," *Virus Evol.*, 4(1), 2018, doi: 10.1093/ve/vex042.

31. Tavakoli, M., Carriere, J., Torabi, A. "Robotics, smart wearable technologies, and autonomous intelligent systems for healthcare during the Covid-19 pandemic: An analysis of the state of the art and future vision," *Adv. Intell. Syst.*, 2(7), 2020, 2000071, doi: https://doi.org/10.1002/aisy.202000071.

32. Nof, S.Y. *Handbook of Industrial Robotics*, 1999. John Wiley & Sons.

33. Hu, Z., Ge, Q., Li, S., Jin, L., Xiong, M. "Artificial intelligence forecasting of Covid-19 in China," *ArXiv200207112 Q-Bio*, Mar. 2020, http://arxiv.org/abs/2002.07112 (accessed: November 21, 2020).

34. Zheng, N. et al. "Predicting Covid-19 in China using hybrid AI model," *IEEE Trans. Cybern.*, 50(7), 2020, 2891–2904, doi: 10.1109/TCYB.2020.2990162.

35. Z. Yang et al. "Modified SEIR and AI prediction of the epidemics trend of Covid-19 in China under public health interventions," *J. Thorac. Dis.*, 12(3), 2020, doi: 10.21037/jtd.2020.02.64.

36. Yang, G.Z. et al. "Combating Covid-19-The role of robotics in managing public health and infectious diseases," *Sci. Robot.*, 5(40), 2020, eabb5589, doi: 10.1126/scirobotics.abb5589.

37. He, W., Zhang, Z. (Justin), Li, W. "Information technology solutions, challenges, and suggestions for tackling the Covid-19 pandemic," *Int. J. Inf. Manag.*, 57, 2021, p. 102287, doi: 10.1016/j.ijinfomgt.2020.102287.

38. "Coronavirus France: Cameras to monitor masks and social distancing," *BBC News*, May 4, 2020, www.bbc.com/news/world-europe-52529981 (accessed: November 21, 2020).

39. ABC News. "How Russia is using facial recognition to police its coronavirus lockdown," *ABC News*, 2020, https://abcnews.go.com/International/russia-facial-recognition-police-coronavirus-lockdown/story?id=70299736 (accessed November 21, 2020).

40. Jain, N. "How Trust In Robots Can Help Us Fight The Next Pandemic," *Forbes*, 2020, www.forbes.com/sites/neerajain/2020/05/20/how-trust-in-robots-can-help-us-fight-the-next-pandemic/ (accessed December 25, 2020).

41. Baidu. "How coronavirus is accelerating a future with autonomous vehicles," *MIT Technology Review*, 2020, www.technologyreview.com/2020/05/18/1001760/how-coronavirus-is-accelerating-autonomous-vehicles/ (accessed December 25, 2020).

42. Nguyen, T.T., Abdelrazek, M., Nguyen, D.T., Aryal, S., Nguyen, D.T., Khatami, A. "Origin of Novel Coronavirus (Covid-19): A computational biology study using artificial intelligence," *bioRxiv*, Jul. 2020, 2020.05.12.091397, doi: 10.1101/2020.05.12.091397.

43. Nguyen, T.T. et al. "Genomic mutations and changes in protein secondary structure and solvent accessibility of SARS-CoV-2 (Covid-19 Virus)," *bioRxiv*, Jul. 2020, 2020.07.10.171769, doi: 10.1101/2020.07.10.171769.

44. Senior, A.W. et al. "Improved protein structure prediction using potentials from deep learning," *Nature*, 577(7792), art. no. 7792, Jan. 2020, doi: 10.1038/s41586-019-1923-7.

45. Zhavoronkov, A. et al. "Potential Covid-2019 3C-like protease inhibitors designed using generative deep learning approaches," Feb. 2020, doi: 10.26434/chemrxiv.11829102.v2.

46. Nguyen, D.D., Gao, K., Chen, J., Wang, R., Wei, G.-W. "Potentially highly potent drugs for 2019-nCoV," *bioRxiv*, Feb. 2020, p. 2020.02.05.936013, doi: 10.1101/2020.02.05.936013.

47. P. Richardson et al. "Baricitinib as potential treatment for 2019-nCoV acute respiratory disease," *The Lancet*, 395(10223), Feb. 2020, e30–e31, doi: 10.1016/S0140-6736(20)30304-4.

10 IoT-Based Healthcare Monitoring Practices during Covid-19

Prospects and Approaches

Safaa N. Saud Al-Humairi and Asif Iqbal Hajamydeen
Faculty of Information Sciences and Engineering
Management and Science University

CONTENTS

The coronavirus outbreak (Covid-19) has led to the declaration of a global pandemic by the World Health Organization (WHO) transforming lifestyle in general. Major sectors of the world's industry and its economy were affected; even the system and management of the Internet of Things (IoT) is not exempted from this. Therefore, this chapter presents an up-to-date survey on the influence of a global pandemic like

DOI: 10.1201/9781003146087-13

Covid-19 on IoT technologies and its environment. It discusses the contributions of IoT and associated sensor technologies in tracing, monitoring, and preventing the virus spread. Consequently, in this chapter, the difficulties in deploying sensor hardware amidst rapidly spreading infections are also addressed. The implications of the global pandemic on the evolution of IoT architectures and infrastructure management is also reviewed, impacting potential effects for prospective IoT implementation. Moreover, it primarily extends insight into the development of sensor-based e-health in managing the global pandemic and determines the issue and impact of a worldwide pandemic that has influenced IoT's future.

10.1 INTRODUCTION

In the advancement of healthcare monitoring and clinical intervention, real-time monitoring systems have significant effects. Patient monitoring systems are the leading mobile health service that supports patients to monitor their vital signs in their daily lives [1]. In e-health, many innovations have recently been implemented to include flexible real-time clinical solutions, such as IoT, cloud computing, and fog computing [2]. These solutions improve business by lowering costs and solving various clinical problems by facilitating multiple operations such as physical and biomedical parameter sensing, processing, and transmission [3]. Regardless of age, gender, location, or health, the objective that presents well-being is to provide autonomous, comfortable, and healthy living. However, age, illness, medications, hospitalisation, epidemics, pandemics, and other conditions are limited.

Health surveillance technologies have been developed to enable healthcare providers and patients to live safely, interact better for closer follow-up, calculate critical health criteria, consult routine, or live healthier generally [4]. In addition, the recent success of ICT on the internet has resulted in smart health supervision and support networks increasing and being able to improve their performance using IoT [5].

Zikali [6] has shown an exponential rise in patients requiring health monitoring. The same investigation estimates that by 2045 the number of seniors viewed as the most disadvantaged in society would be greater than young adults and children. Yet, there is a shortage of domestic healthcare staff, caregivers, and physicians worldwide, ensuring that care is costly for senior-aged adults. Surveillance of the healthcare system [7] may play a crucial part in reducing a patient's physical movement, stay in the hospital, appointment times, waiting lists, and general health costs while reducing medical personnel's workload, stress, and burden [8]. The expansion of the dominant health systems in telemedicine applications and portrait health networks contributes to ICT advancement for communication to be ubiquitous [9].

In addition to clinics, hospitals, or other containment facilities, introducing smart home technology offers safe living and enhanced quality of the care of the elderly, the disabled for an independent and comfortable life [10, 11]. The medical module can boost health services for patients at home or remote areas (infrequent reachability to hospitals) in the sense of an intelligent home automation system. Depression in hospital wards is reduced by patients' isolation [12]. Doctors can monitor patients in their offices and prescribe remote diagnostic medicine and show the basic parameters of measured health. The rapid improvement of intelligent home healthcare software and hardware allows users, particularly elderly and handicapped individuals, to easily track home appliances from smartphones, tablets, and laptops [13].

An intelligent home healthcare environment comprises various computer devices that work on behalf of users and thus render such an ecosystem all-round. User context and preferences in a smart home healthcare environment are vital to decision making, such that patients can select between resources and services [14]. The context-conscious paradigm provides perception into domestic aspects affecting physiological readings' output [15]. Any information that may clarify an entity's (person) state regarding its physiological health status or needs is the user context. IoT's four dynamic functional components record, transfer, analyse, and process data. Data can be obtained using sensors attached to mobile devices like tablets, robots, and health monitoring systems for end-users. In this scenario, system maintenance is needed to avoid any potential malfunctions. Patient evaluation and data analysis are necessary for transmitting collected data to the cloud server for decision-making and analysis [16].

IoT applications in the medical sector have been applied to different networks such as medical devices, cloud computing, large-format data, cloud computing, pharmaceutical systems, and other application types [17]. For the combat against Covid-19, it is possible to apply IoT technologies to various healthcare field users, for example, remote patient surveillance, remote communication network tracking, and manual sensor-based monitoring systems [18–20].

10.2 ADOPTION APPEARANCE OF THE HOSPITAL TECHNOLOGIES

The IoT-based network of architectural systems and artefacts facilitates the study, perception, and control of remote healthcare delivery devices [21]. For information processing in the IoT architecture, the network system mainly relies on the middleware layer. IoT's fundamental architecture consists of three levels of perception, transmission, and implementation, which are then expanded to include different architectures in the middleware and business levels [22]. The three-layer IoT core architecture (Figure 10.1) provides perception, transmission, and application layers to different middleware and business layers [23].

(1) The perception layer is defined as sensor devices, and their objective matters can detect and recognise the object and collect data for further processing in the next layer.

(2) Transmission layer: the relation between servers, network devices, and intelligent objects is a crucial part of this layer. The sensors' data will be transferred from the perception layer into the middleware layer through the 3G network, wireless, LAN, RFID Bluetooth, and vice versa.

(3) Middleware layer: is often named the processing layer and stores massive quantities of information from the transmission layer. It oversees database access and services management and links it to the cloud with considerable data processing information.

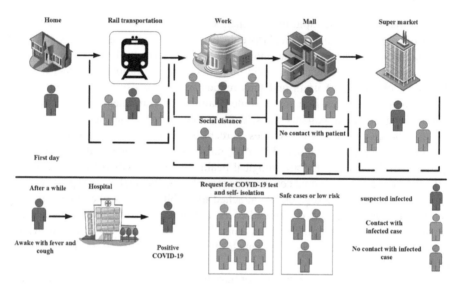

FIGURE 10.1   IoT monitoring and tracing platform architecture [23].

(4) Application layer: this layer provides end-users with application-oriented services. End-users will have interacted directly with this layer by allowing application layer protocols.

(5) Business layer: This is a well-designed, successful business model; the business layer manages the entire IoT ecosystem, permitting the end consumer to make more actionable decisions.

10.3   ADOPTION OF IOT TECHNOLOGIES FOR HEALTHCARE PERSISTENCE

The main advances in designing intelligent home mechanisation technology and e-health systems permit citizens to benefit as home medical assistants without hospitalisation [24]. Mobile patient health monitoring through home health technology enables healthcare providers, medical staff, and doctors to access patients without physical or hospital contact. Healthcare technologies regularly save patients costs and discomfort by avoiding physical contact to meet their healthcare providers or medical staff [25]. Many types of research have been published in intelligent health, e-health, and distance care [3, 26, 27].

A framework for e-health tracking patients in handling critical physical parameters from any position was proposed by the authors [28]. The system collected and was made accessible and visible to the physician with essential data of the patient. The web application offers to store data, drug advisory notes, medication and dose for the patient while allowing them to obtain fundamental parameter values on psychological metrics and display the doctor's information [29, 30]. Every day, the intelligent mobile application reminded patients of their treatments, medications, and other

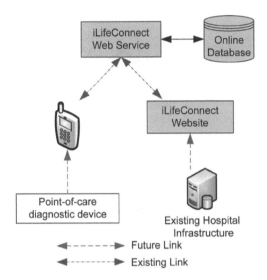

FIGURE 10.2   The architecture of the system [33].

activities. Finally, a mobile application has the same functionality as a web application and has an additional link from a different location and at any time [31].

As an apprentice for the blood pressure measurement via the mobile application, a remote health surveillance system was introduced by Sparsh and Chiew [32]. The collected values on mobile apps were triggered and displayed via the system's web interface to doctors or caregivers. Healthcare professionals and specialist doctors will track, manage, and send feedback to the patient through the designed system accordingly. The authors in [33], the Body Sensor Network (BSN), shown in Figure 10.2, proposed a healthy and up-to-date IoT health monitoring system. The method suggested tests and tracks physiology such as blood pressure via electrocardiograms and wearable body sensors. The patient's data is processed in the BSN-Care server database for analysis. The system notifies family member, the nearest physician, or the patient movement in the emergency room, depending on the test and the malformation's condition. A lightweight anonymous authentication protocol is used to ensure the BSN-Care server users' identification. The Offset Codebook (OCB) Encoding scheme has been used to protect anonymity, data integrity, and data input.

Minh Pham et al. [34] introduced a cloud-based smart home environment (CoSHE) for a wearable home healthcare unit (see Figure 10.3a), private cloud, and robot helpers. A CoSHE device gathers comprehensive non-invasive wearable sensors from residents. It provides information on everyday operations and their location in the house, as shown in the home interior design in Figure 10.3b. A web application that builds on the system's cloud server offers detailed health data for caregivers. The device also has an application for hydration control to monitor the patient's water intake and daily fluid requirement. Hydration monitors are carried out using acoustic

(a)

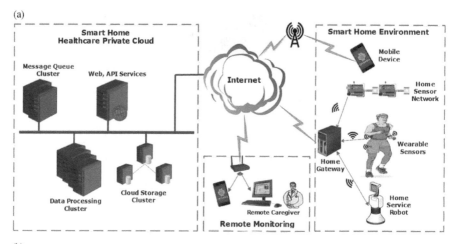

(b)

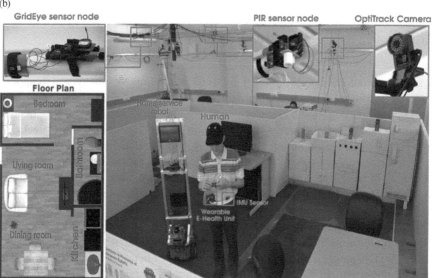

FIGURE 10.3   (a) Cloud-based smart home healthcare system architecture and (b) The smart home testbed [34].

data gathered from a smartwatch accelerometer's microphones and body activity background.

Eren Demir [35] has presented a smart home framework controlled by an Android operating system strengthening the environment for persons with dementia. The device architecture makes it possible to store, record, and transmit data via a cloud application. The platform comprises seven sensors for identifying a person's movement or current position, flame detection, and use of Minh Pham et al. [34], a CoSHE that includes a private cloud, home health wearable unit, and a computerised robot helper. CoSHE collects extensive wearable sensors as non-invasive units from residents and offers a report on day-to-day activities. Comprehensive health data will then be sent to specialist doctors and healthcare professionals via mobile or web applications.

Eren Demir [35] has presented a mobile application android based that works as an integrated smart home framework to support the ecosystem for persons with dementia. Device architecture makes it possible to store, record, and transfer the data via the cloud application. The device consists of seven sensors function with a standing or seated mode to identify flame, and the use of various domestic appliances. The sensors often inform or warn the patient about certain things, whether they forget to do them in time. To detect whether or not the light is on, a button is also mounted on the device. It also helps recognise patients' behaviours and provide the doctor or caregiver with information. Data is obtained from various sensors installed for processing in specific locations at home.

Bilal and Khaled [36] recommended that an old, handicapped, decrepit, and disabled wireless home automation system be installed. The unit was designed to be very compact to make it easier to operate and track patients with locomotor difficulties of vital home appliances. System users can monitor or track devices using XBee technology, which sends messages to receivers connected to different electronic devices. Remote control features include control buttons for various devices and LCD alerts. A wood prototype version was added to the proposed system. Min Chen et al. [37] suggested a second-generation RFID management framework for e-health, illustrated in Figure 10.4. Through a video conferencing call, the patient can communicate with the on-call doctor or another health professional. The video call is made with the system's protection as a backup to the on-call doctor. The device can also gather and turn knowledge in the care of medical emergencies. The sensor will be directly contacted to the patient's body to retrieve physiological signals, including heart rate, temperature, and blood rate. The device also has a digital database to track users and their medical records.

To acquire users' health condition and propose actions, Andrea et al. [38] developed an improved sensing technique based on an integrated sensor network to monitor homes and living environments. The authors propose a platform that includes sensors to monitor physiological elements such as electrocardiogram (ECG), cardiac velocity, breathing rate, blood pressure, biomedical, wearable, and non-transparent.

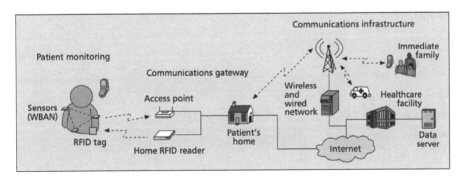

FIGURE 10.4   A 2G-RFID-enabled e-healthcare system [37].

The mobile-sensor interfacing was designed as a mobile application. The information, including responses and demographic information, is forwarded to the cloud for storage and data analyses for various elderly-related purposes. After some experimentation with a user-friendly home app architecture. Abdelsalam et al. [39] designed clinical software that has built a successful way for patients to follow their blood sugar levels. The framework in Figure 10.5a aims to track patient behaviours, diet, and compliance utilising personal connected devices and intelligent home technology to assess the impact of alternative medicines and regimens. For access to technology in the architecture, wearable devices are used. Data created by wearable devices and intelligent spaces are massive, representing thousands of readings each day, as demonstrated in Figure 10.5b on the Atlas sensor platform [40].

Muhammad et al. [41] have created an Android mobile application for the elderly, independent of their homes. The application records and manages users' everyday activities and acts as reminders of the patient's expected job. The system also offers warnings when operations are incomplete, meaningful, and ignored. The system

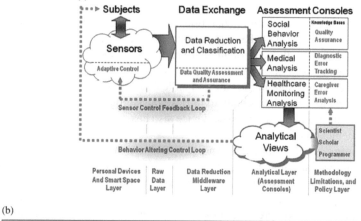

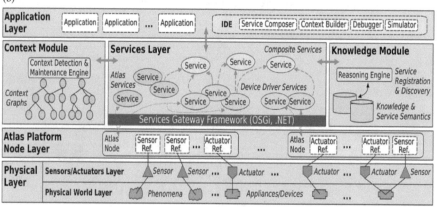

FIGURE 10.5 (a) Health platform architecture and (b) Atlas middleware [39].

also monitors humidity, gas leakage, and temperature as a complete environmental scanning. The recorded information from the continuous patient monitoring will be provided to family members and healthcare professionals for a better monitoring and following of current status if needed. As for the system's activities to address the needs of older adults for continued treatment, Hossain et al. [42] suggested a smart home health system focused on an ecosystem in intelligent cities (Figure 10.6). Inputs to the proposed interface (dialogue and video) are numerous to monitor patients' well-being. Data from camera sensors and microphones are continuously collected, transmitted to a particular cloud for processing, and the graduation results are produced. Physicians prescribe and serve performance-based on the classification ratings through audio and video messages.

Saiteja et al. [43] proposed a smart home health system to monitor diabetes and blood pressure wirelessly. To keep the healthcare professional up to date with any irregularities and avoid high pressure and diabetes in patients through preparation, the computer analyses the blood pressure and glucose readings accordingly. The supporting vector machine classifier was used to perform successful and efficient training activities. Furthermore, the device will give a licensed physician clinic

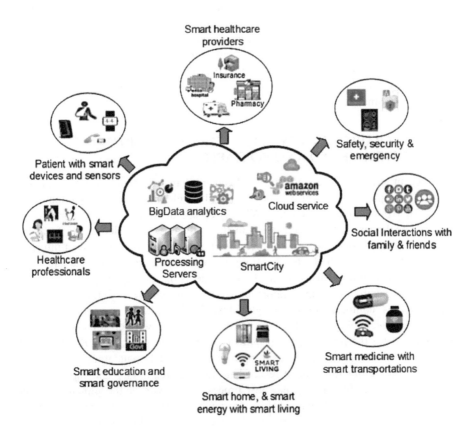

FIGURE 10.6   Smart health in the smart city ecosystem [42].

warnings and real-time updates of patient health from their home. In an Android platform, Kashif et al. [44] have built an intelligent home technology (IPC) framework for seniors. The system has been designed to enhance the elderly quality of life, avoid electrical waste, and, at the same time, preserve people's energy through remote access. The device also tracks environmental criteria based on senior citizens' health and living standards and triggers warnings when their homes are disturbed and disrupted.

10.4   E-HEALTHCARE TECHNOLOGIES FOR PRE-COVID-19 DIAGNOSIS

MobiHealthNews announced in January 2020 that the Shanghai Public Health Center (SPHCC) used VivaLNK's uninterrupted temperature sensor for tracking Covid-19 patients, based on a linked California-based healthcare start-up to minimise the risks of carers being exposed to this virus [45]. Recently, SPHCC and VivaLNK Medical Wearables have announced their use of Bluetooth IoT gateways and solutions providers for Covid-19 patients.

The gateways in Cassia are used to receive patient information in real time from sensors and relay this data wirelessly for continuous monitoring at a nurse station. The medical personnel's vital network management tool is Cassia's access IoT controller, used to track patients and provide an overview of their lives in real time. Cassia gateways permit the simultaneous pairing and connection of up to 40 Bluetooth Low Energy devices while offering the long-range connectivity required for the SPHCC in several rooms. Cassias gateways are being used for the SPHCC and seven other hospitals in China [46].

10.5   WEARABLE DEVICES VS HEALTHCARE MONITORING SYSTEMS: FIXED AND PORTABLE

Over recent years, this technology has been used in healthcare and clinical trial settings anticipating the level of innovation and development in wearable technologies [47]. Work-based assessments (WBAS) can be defined as a front portion that encloses healthcare data unobtrusively in the body. WBAS collects data from the body through embedded sensors through direct or indirect means to collect information from the patient's body. Furthermore, it prepares data for either onboard input or remote transmission for robust analytic and decision-making support. Moreover, the usage of health monitoring equipment in clinical research is a significant factor in certain studies' continuity during the global pandemic [48].

Wearable technology products, initially developed with customers in mind, have created for the pharmaceutical industry a world of opportunity. Relaxed FDA regulations on monitoring needs resulting from the Covid-19 pandemic [49] will provide more flexibility for clinical researchers to meet regulatory and reporting criteria and enhance the participants' test process. Forecasts of the global wearable healthcare market have shown substantial growth for several years, and the demand in the middle of 2019 showed a potential market of $139.4 billion in 2026, up from $24.6 billion in 2018. Clinical science is now shifting paradigms since this growth in mobile health (mHealth) powered by customers offers a way to continue operations within budgetary and logistical constraints. More decentralised clinical trials, trial supervisors communicating less with patients, wearables, and remote collection technologies are becoming ever more useful for completing studies [50].

In Munich, Cosinuss® offers the ground-breaking biosensor technology to track low- and mid-risk patients living in home isolation from Covid-19. Cosinuss provides a cost-efficient, easy-to-use workbench for healthcare centres and can be configured quickly with the monitoring system. It consists of a wearable in-ear sensor, a data gateway, a Cosinuss LabApp, and the servers (Cosinuss LabServer) [45]. The in-ear sensor gathers the main physiological parameters from the isolated patient. It transmits the data to the Cosinuss server, which calculates the compound score in real time with early warning algorithms. All critical patient information can be obtained via a simple web interface by health professionals. The Cosinuss solution allows medical professionals to focus on the need for hospital admission and the urgency of their respective health conditions.

Like most medical equipment, the primary physiological monitoring parameters are core body temperature, air velocity, blood oxygen saturation, and heart rate. The wearable in-ear sensor and a Cosinusso gateway are given for low- to medium-risk patients. The wearable sensor monitors vital sign data inside the ear channel (see Figure 10.7a) and sends the collected values to the data gateway via Bluetooth 4.0. A mobile application (Cosinusso LabApp) or an autonomous computer may capture and store data. The patient's data passage from here transmits the data obtained to the Cosinuss LabServer in real time or fixed. The collected vital information in the LabServer is processed in real time, employing advanced algorithms and analyses to assess the early warning results. Through the Cosinuss Web Interface (Figure 10.7b), healthcare professionals can imagine and access critical patient information. Researchers may use a standard GUI to access the anonymised health data of the LabServer. The Cosinuss° LabServer integrates a cloud database with a web interface that provides health centres with reliable data and the ability to monitor patients remotely [51]. The server's extra processing capacity allows data analysis in real time [52]. Advanced algorithms measure additional primary physiological parameters, including breathing speed and variability in heart rate.

10.6   COVID-19 UTILISES ADOPTION IOT IN HOSPITALS

Given the pressure on hospital resources, patients' monitoring tools offer substantial relief for various healthcare facilities to deliver service effectively. Monitoring instruments permit health workers to remotely provide their services without arriving at each patient's particular location. This remote monitoring system also offers medical practitioners and nursing staff extensive assistance, especially in the hospital environment, reducing the required physical efforts.

In combating disease, the value of general clean-up has become essential and is spreading further in public facilities. As a result of the current global pandemic, multiple IoT-based solutions were created to assist workers' health. Hospitals in Vancouver, Canada, for instance, are installing battery-powered IoT buttons by Wanda Quicktouch, a warning of maintenance and cleaning problems that could

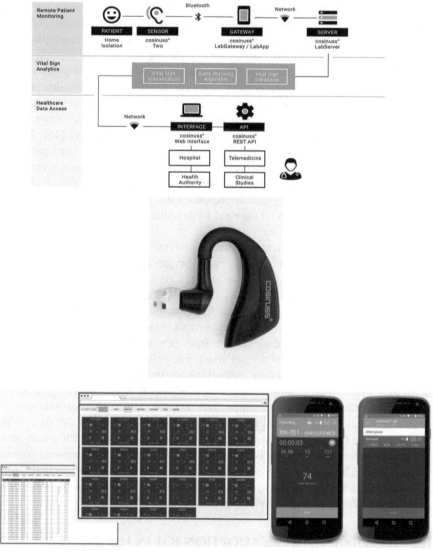

FIGURE 10.7 (a)   Wearable in-ear sensor and cosinusso-gateway and (b) Cosinuss° Web and mobile interfaces [51].

pose a safety threat to the public [53]. In the Central Militar Hospital in Mexico, a centre has been established to attend Covid-19 patients during the pandemic without failing to participate in other emergencies [54] as shown in the schematic approach in Figure 10.8.

As pandemic spreads rapidly among the masses, the vital signs of patients' monitoring are essential in delivering health services. Because of its infectious existence, any interaction between medical practitioners and patients to determine the

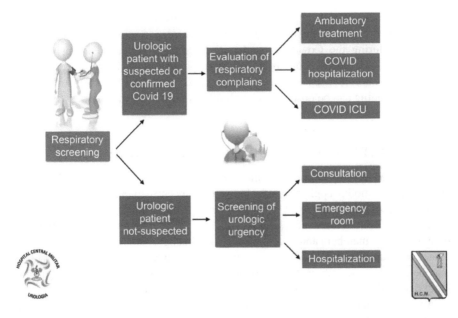

FIGURE 10.8 Approach patients with suspected urological emergency or confirmed diagnosis of Covid-19 [54].

patient's body temperature raises the risk of Covid-19 being contracted by the medical professional. A specific device has been set up in some hospitals with an Aranet PRO10 base station and bacteria-controlled wireless body temperature sensors [55] to solve this issue. Aranet Medical Thermometer with multi-sensors wirelessly transmits the measured data to the central monitoring device as a reading per minute and consequently alerts medical doctors or health takers if any medical treatment is needed and provides an accessible patient history.

It is crucial to safely track and care for the sickest patients in the face of challenging the Covid-19 pandemic spreading with insufficient ICU beds, services, and healthcare staff. The imminent crisis provides innovation opportunities in which the pandemic will lead to the development and innovation of a normally slow-moving healthcare system. The use of remote technologies in managing the influx of critically ill patients with Covid-19 can relieve the healthcare burden and reduce exposure to Covid-19 from healthcare providers. However, its use should be strengthened by data safety and cybersecurity. It is imperative to have better patient treatment round the clock. An ICU remote-tracking technique was developed using cameras and smartphones using CCTV (closed-circuit television). High-definition CCTV cameras were mounted over each ICU bed to view the patient mechanical ventilation and monitoring system all around the clock. A CCTV system was reported analogous to an audio-visual doffing system controlled from location to location to improve personnel safety [56]. It is a mobile health monitoring module and a server structure. The smartphone shows essential patient parameters such as temperature, SpO2, ECG, heart rate, blood pressure, O$_2$ percentage, and respiratory rate. The professional is aided in tracking, alerting, and handling patient treatment without being present on the night [57] with a flexible, agile, and cost-effective remote ICU surveillance technology during the Covid-19 pandemic. Second, experienced intensivists can track several ICU patients' conditions on a smartphone remotely. Thirdly, continuous physiological surveillance is provided 24 hours a day. Finally, earlier than unexpected clinical worsening can be observed, and clinicians on-site may be advised to mediate in good time.

10.7   SMART HEALTHCARE MONITORING SYSTEMS

The integrated development environment of Android Studio was used to design and create Android mobile applications for home appliances, medical devices, and doctor-in-home communications [44]. Users can access the mobile application by registering with the application; after successful registration, the user can log in as a patient and monitor family members and access profiles and background based on the submitted data. For future purposes, user registers for domestic devices and additional widgets may be added. As sensors irritate the patient's body, this programme includes manual input data and cannot automatically measure physiological conditions.

A user should use the health parameter before measuring the automated collection of health data. The mobile application's health interface allows the user to do tasks such as chatting, leave a message, or check for medicines prescribed by the doctor. The mobile application can also communicate Covid-19 findings to your doctor, mainly when the patient follows obligatory home or government self-isolation quarantine. Intervals are observed and tested for the relevant symptoms. The readings are sent to the doctor, and an answer is obtained once the value and responses to the Covid-19 symptoms have been successfully reported. This program is designed to evaluate the incoming inputs and answer the patient's next action [40]. The red colour sign means that the patient must report immediately to the nearest hospital or Covid-19 centre; orange indicates that the patient shows over 80% of Covid-19 symptoms; yellow suggests that the patient experiences too mild symptoms to exhibit the same effect. The feedback indicates a moderate sign and the patient's appropriate intervention. The doctor will advise and prescribe the needed medicines based on the criteria obtained at the end of the doctor consultation.

Remote patient monitoring for home control of Covid-19 in New York was designed by Laura Tabacof et al. [58]. This application can monitor regular physiologic data and symptom intensity on the patients, as shown in Figure 10.9. Furthermore, details about comorbidity (i.e., is the presence of one or more additional conditions often co-occurring (i.e., concomitant or concurrent with) with a primary condition) and Covid-19 test results were given during the referral process. If the Platelet-rich plasma (PRP) practitioner was accredited as clinically suggested, the patient's inpatient appointment was scheduled by a clinician. During the onboarding process, each patient had to download software applications such as Electronic Data Capture (REDCap) and MyCap. Patients were provided with a manual that included descriptions of program usage and specific guidance on filling out the forms.

In addition, patients deemed by their prescribing physician or PRP clinician to be at high risk of rapid respiratory decline were fitted with a pulse oximeter. Criteria

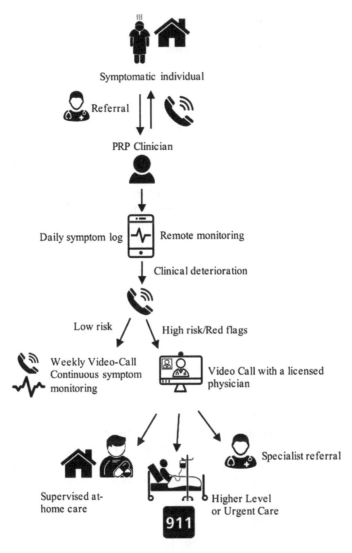

FIGURE 10.9 Precision recovery workflow diagram [58].

suggesting an increased risk of respiratory deterioration include: individuals with a medical history of respiratory severe or cardiovascular disease, individuals with supplemental oxygen discharge from the inpatient setting, or those with complicated patient stays, including those requiring mechanical ventilation or acute respiratory failure, and patients with severe Covid-19 symptoms.

10.8 BIOMETRIC MONITORING TECHNOLOGIES

There are various BioMeTs available remotely to capture vital signs for Covid-19 and patient care, such as temperature, heart rate, BP, and blood oxygen saturation (SpO2).

One reason that did not include disclosure-related symptoms as diagnostic-related symptoms for each concept is that the symptoms associated with each measurement definition are subjective and vary over time.

10.8.1 Body Temperature

In Covid-19, fever in between 50 and 87% of patients on hospital admission is a typical but variable symptom. Continuous real-time temperature monitoring provides improved possibilities of tracking improvements in asymptomatic patients or those with moderate symptoms at home [59]. The thermo-resistors are based on the resistance concept, the ease of electricity flowing through metal, and direct contact with the body for measurement. The heat of a metal increases strength, and an algorithm measures temperature resistance fluctuation. Thermophiles BioMeTs as Infrared thermometers based used to calculate thermal radiation intensity from the surface and does not required a direct contact with the body [60, 61].

10.8.2 Heart Rate

There are several reasons for high basal heart rates or changes in the heart rhythm, which can be seen in infected patients. Studies decide how improvements will predict and track Covid-19 progression in cardiac rates and heart rate variability [61]. Two sensor modalities are frequently used in BioMeTs to measure heart rhythm, cardiac defects using ECGs and photoplethysmography (PPGs). Often track ECGs are used to test electricity in the heart using electrodes, and several trackers are used for customer fitness with PPG, also known as heart rate optical sensors [62]. A PPG uses light to measure blood volume pulses, which means that the number of lights that move through the skin affects the blood volume. By measuring the time between changes in the blood flow, the light sensor measures the heart rate. Although ECG is a traditional standard for comprehensive cardiovascular research, including cardiovascular diagnosis and classification, PPG is a convenient tool for detecting cardiovascular events [63].

10.8.3 Blood Pressure

In hospitalised patients with Covid-19, hypertension was found to be common comorbidity. In patients who died of Covid-19, a higher incidence of hypertension than in survivors was recorded. Unlike other vital signs, remote BP monitoring has well-established product validation procedures and generally accepted recommendations for particular patient groups and environments, including clinical, ambulatory, or home environments [64]. The high prevalence of hypertension in adults, which requires a regular evaluation of patient conditions, drives these rigorous procedures. Remote BP monitoring for white-coat hypertension and masked hypertension is an essential clinical care delivery [65]. BioMeTs permit data to be collected over extended periods to understand BP-change trends that cannot be identified during visits to a clinic office (for example, continued, white-coat, masked and nightly hypertension). Technical organisations have developed formal product validation procedures. In the peer-review literature or on validation websites, lists of goods tested by independent parties are available. Furthermore, there are recommendations for product preference in some cases, such as home care, paediatric measurements, or obesity measurements in patients [66].

10.8.4 BLOOD OXYGEN SATURATION (SPO2)

A patient's SpO2 and respiratory rate are routinely measured when determining their mechanical ventilation needs. Various air and heart diseases, including Covid-19, can result in low SpO2. Low SpO2 was found in Covid-19 to be linked to poor performance [67]. Individual patients with Covid-19, who have no respiratory distress and a hazardously low oxygen level, are considered quiet hypoxemia. The use of pulse oximeters in the home will help patients remotely triage and can help classify patients who can seek medical advice and treatment in a personal setting earlier [68].

10.8.5 RESPIRATORY RATE

Respiratory rate (RR) is a significant indicator of respiratory distress. Elevated RR can be observed on arrival, usually correlated with bad outcomes. Traditional medical tests are unreliable and prone to error for continuous monitoring. Infrared cameras also assess pulse and respiratory rate by observing chest wall movement or cardiac activity [69, 70].

10.9 SELF-MONITORING DEVICES BASED ON IOT IN COVID-19 APPLICATIONS

Figure 10.10 introduces a generic IoT-based self-monitoring system consisting of various sensors, communication, and controls. In addition, IoT device-based medical homes are currently employed in enhancing outpatient care and reducing hospital visits. There are also benefits for drug failure during a pandemic because of medical home-fitted mobile devices [71]. IoT-dependent drug management effectively reduces the burden on medical personnel. This approach allows healthcare professionals to access patients' daily information by connecting it with their medical records.

It is an integral part of keeping a routine medicine schedule. Maintaining an acceptable regimen of medication is most critical under all circumstances. When the medical system is stretched beyond its limits, maintaining medical affairs within the family provides substantial relief. IoT equipment and techniques have been applied to combat the Covid-19 pandemic outbreak [72]. A self-monitoring system focused on IoT has minimised the spread of the Covid-19 pandemic. An application allows people to contribute and access different types of information, allowing them to work with the government in developing the country. The citizen application enable users to track if they are quarantined.

10.10 IMPACT OF IOT APPLICATIONS ON MITIGATING THE SPREAD OF COVID-19

The integrated network for the efficient transaction and sharing of data is the core element of IoT, which is valuable for both citizens and benefactors. Using the proposed IoT tactic in the Covid-19 pandemic, a greater degree of traceability for

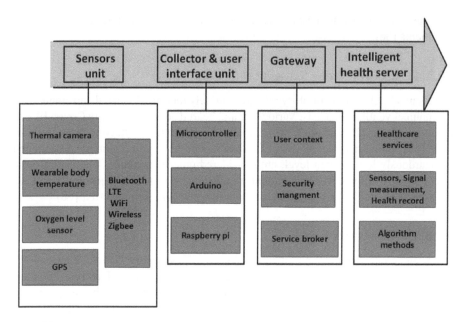

FIGURE 10.10   A generic framework for self-monitoring based IoT system [71].

patients can be attained. By developing a well-informed community of individuals or organisations into a linked network, cluster identification can be more successful [73]. By implementing smart technology to provide physical therapy services, hospitals can relieve mental stress and improve comfort levels. Research conducted at MIT showed that the geo-encoded data from personal health trackers and cell phones could be used to locate the source of a virus outbreak. Implementing this technology can also help treat patients with health problems [74].

10.11   BENEFITS FOR CLINICAL RESEARCHERS

Despite the difficulties of mHealth, biometry from wearable medical devices may provide researchers with many qualitative and functional advantages for healthcare systems when used in single-blinded studies [75, 76], including:

- Precise remote control of participants with digital data, remove clinical site visits and facilitate studies in the absence of global or local unexpected catastrophes.
- A more realistic, real world view of a patient's reaction with ongoing health surveillance and response to a test drug than patient-reported anecdotal evidence.
- Preceding decision-making by providing almost continuing real-time data access. For instance, researchers can change protocols based on how participants respond in real time to a drug.
- Specific intervention allows researchers to alert themselves to possible adverse events or patient loss earlier during the experiment.

- Improve the retention of subjects by presenting and sharing information to facilitate active patient engagement.
- Reduced cost by minimising the length and cost of clinic visits and precise and comprehensive monitoring of the patients despite decentralised trials.
- Mobile sensor data can provide additional information to researchers to demonstrate the advantages of a drug, opening the potential for different research approaches.
- Both data points can be obtained safely and remotely so that trials can proceed smoothly, irrespective of the situation, using wearables and other home monitoring supplies.

10.12 CONCLUSION

IoT in healthcare is directed to a significant advancement in mobile healthcare and improved social lifestyle, primarily for senior citizens. Merging home automation with healthcare systems has relieved stress, lowered the cost of living and facilitated remote interaction among patients and doctors. The chapter has presented a recent review on the impact of a global pandemic on IoT technologies. IoT and related sensor technologies' contributions in tracking, examining, and thwarting the virus spread were discussed. Subsequently, the difficulties in implementing sensor hardware during the pandemic were also addressed. The implications of the global pandemic on the evolution of IoT architectures and infrastructure management were also reviewed. Moreover, the development of sensor-based e-health in managing the worldwide pandemic and the concern and influence of a global pandemic on the future of IoT has been elaborated.

REFERENCES

1. Gómez, J., Oviedo, B., Zhuma, E. "Patient monitoring system based on internet of things", *Procedia Computer Science*, 83, 2016, 90–97.
2. Al Nuaimi, N. et al. "e-Health cloud implementation issues and efforts," in *International Conference on Industrial Engineering and Operations Management (IEOM)*, 2015. IEEE.
3. Rahmani, A.M. et al. "Exploiting smart e-Health gateways at the edge of healthcare Internet-of-Things: A fog computing approach," *Future Generation Computer Systems*, 78, 2018, 641–658.
4. Dang, L.M., et al. "A survey on internet of things and cloud computing for healthcare," *Electronics*, 8(7), 2019, 768.
5. Zhan, K. "Sports and health big data system based on 5G network and Internet of Things system," *Microprocessors and Microsystems*, 2020, 103363.
6. Zikali, Z. "Health-E news.No Suitable Care for SA's Elderly," 22, 2018.
7. Al-Humairi, S.N.S., Kamal, A.A.A. "Design a smart infrastructure monitoring system: a response in the age of Covid-19 pandemic," *Innovative Infrastructure Solutions*, 6(3), 2021, 1–10.
8. Mphande, T. *A secure patient monitoring and tracking system using RFID and internet of things for the university teaching hospital*, 2020. University of Zambia.
9. Bedekar, H., Hossain, G., Goyal, A. "Medical Analytics Based on Artificial Neural Networks Using Cognitive Internet of Things," in *Fog Data Analytics for IoT Applications*, 2020. Springer. pp. 199–262.

10. Lim, W.S. et al. "COVID-19 and Older People in Asia: AWGS Calls to Actions," *Geriatrics & Gerontology International*, 2020.

11. Agustina, R. et al. "Universal health coverage in Indonesia: concept, progress, and challenges," *The Lancet*, 393(10166), 2019, 75–102.

12. Albahri, O. et al. "Real-time remote health-monitoring Systems in a Medical Centre: A review of the provision of healthcare services-based body sensor information, open challenges and methodological aspects," *Journal of Medical Systems*, 42(9), 2018, 164.

13. Katuk, N. et al. "Implementation and recent progress in cloud-based smart home automation systems," in *2018 IEEE Symposium on Computer Applications & Industrial Electronics (ISCAIE)*, 2018. IEEE.

14. Boivin, A. et al. "Involving patients in setting priorities for healthcare improvement: a cluster randomised trial," *Implementation Science*, 9(1), 2014, 24.

15. Yang, Q. "A novel recommendation system based on semantics and context awareness," *Computing*, 100(8), 2018, 809–823.

16. Gia, T.N. et al. "IoT-based continuous glucose monitoring system: A feasibility study," *Procedia Computer Science*, 109, 2017, 327–334.

17. Sousa, P.R., Antunes, L., Martins, R. "The present and future of privacy-preserving computation in fog computing," in *Fog Computing in the Internet of Things*, 2018. Springer. p. 51–69.

18. Ndiaye, M. et al. "IoT in the wake of Covid-19: A survey on contributions, challenges and evolution," *IEEE Access*, 8, 2020, 186821–186839.

19. Al-Humairi, S.N.S. et al. "Conceptual Design: A Novel Covid-19 Smart AI Helmet," *Int J Emerg Technol*, 2020, 11(5), 389–396.

20. Al-Humairi, S.N.S., Kamal, A.A.A. "Opportunities and challenges for the building monitoring systems in the age-pandemic of Covid-19: Review and prospects," *Innovative Infrastructure Solutions*, 6(2), 2021, 79.

21. Al-Humairi, S. et al. *Covid-19 PANDEMIC: Monitoring Technologies. Healthcare and Panic buying behaviour*, 2020. White Falcon Publishing.

22. Jia, M. et al. "Adopting Internet of Things for the development of smart buildings: A review of enabling technologies and applications," *Automation in Construction*, 101, 2019, 111–126.

23. Al-Ogaili, A.S. et al. "IoT Technologies for Tackling Covid-19 in Malaysia and Worldwide: Challenges, Recommendations, and Proposed Framework," *Computers, Materials & Continua*, 66(2), 2141–2164.

24. Majumder, S. et al. "Smart homes for elderly healthcare—Recent advances and research challenges," *Sensors*, 17(11), 2017, 2496.

25. Pomey, M.-P. et al. "Patients as partners: a qualitative study of patients' engagement in their health care," *PloS One*, 10(4), 2015, e0122499.

26. Bagula, A. et al. "Cloud based patient prioritisation as service in public health care," in *2016 ITU Kaleidoscope: ICTs for a Sustainable World (ITU WT)*, 2016. IEEE.

27. Khan, S.U. et al. "An e-Health care services framework for the detection and classification of breast cancer in breast cytology images as an IoMT application," *Future Generation Computer Systems*, 98, 2019, 286–296.

28. Aleksandar, K., Natasa, K., Saso, K. "E-health monitoring system," in *International Conference on Applied Internet and Information Technologies*, 2016.

29. Ozdalga, E., Ozdalga, A., Ahuja, N. "The smartphone in medicine: a review of current and potential use among physicians and students," *Journal of Medical Internet Research*, 14(5), 2012, e128.

30. Gravenhorst, F. et al. "Mobile phones as medical devices in mental disorder treatment: an overview," *Personal and Ubiquitous Computing*, 19(2), 2015, 335–353.

31. Micallef, N., Baillie, L., Uzor, S. "Time to exercise! An aide-memoire stroke app for post-stroke arm rehabilitation," in *Proceedings of the 18th international conference on Human-computer interaction with mobile devices and services*, 2016.

32. Agarwal, S., Lau, C.T. "Remote health monitoring using mobile phones and Web services," *Telemedicine and e-Health*, 16(5), 2010, 603–607.

33. Gope, P., Hwang, T. "BSN-Care: A secure IoT-based modern healthcare system using body sensor network," *IEEE sensors journal*, 16(5), 2015, 1368–1376.

34. Pham, M. et al. "Delivering home healthcare through a cloud-based smart home environment (CoSHE)," *Future Generation Computer Systems*, 81, 2018, 129–140.

35. Demir, E. et al. "Smart home assistant for ambient assisted living of elderly people with dementia," *Procedia Computer Science*, 113, 2017, 609–614.

36. Ghazal, B., Al, K. -Khatib, "Smart home automation system for elderly, and handicapped people using XBee," *International Journal of Smart Home*, 9(4), 2015, 203–210.

37. Chen, M. et al. "A 2G-RFID-based e-healthcare system," *IEEE Wireless Communications*, 17(1), 2010, 37–43.

38. Monteriù, A. et al. "A smart sensing architecture for domestic monitoring: methodological approach and experimental validation," *Sensors*, 18(7), 2018, 2310.

39. Helal, A., Cook, D.J., Schmalz, M. "Smart home-based health platform for behavioral monitoring and alteration of diabetes patients," *Journal of Diabetes Science and Technology*, 3(1), 2009, 141–148.

40. Taiwo, O., A.E. Ezugwu, "Smart healthcare support for remote patient monitoring during covid-19 quarantine," *Informatics in Medicine Unlocked*, 20, 2020, 100428.

41. Fahim, M. et al. "Daily life activity tracking application for smart homes using android smartphone," in *2012 14th International conference on advanced communication technology (ICACT)*, 2012. IEEE.

42. Hossain, M.S. "Patient status monitoring for smart home healthcare," in *2016 IEEE International Conference on Multimedia & Expo Workshops (ICMEW)*, 2016. IEEE.

43. Chatrati, S.P. et al. "Smart home health monitoring system for predicting type 2 diabetes and hypertension," *Journal of King Saud University-Computer and Information Sciences*, 2020.

44. Nisar, K. et al. "Smart home for elderly living using Wireless Sensor Networks and an Android application," in *2016 IEEE 10th international conference on application of information and communication technologies (AICT)*, 2016. IEEE.

45. Channa, A., Popescu, N. "Managing Covid-19 Global Pandemic with High-Tech Consumer Wearables: A Comprehensive Review," in *2020 12th International Congress on Ultra Modern Telecommunications and Control Systems and Workshops (ICUMT)*, 2020. IEEE.

46. Sharma, D., Nawab, A.Z.B., Alam, M. "Integrating M-Health with IoMT to Counter Covid-19," in *Computational Intelligence Methods in Covid-19: Surveillance, Prevention, Prediction and Diagnosis*, 2020. Springer. pp. 373–396.

47. Jin, H., Jin, Q., Jian, J. "Smart materials for wearable healthcare devices," *Wearable Technologies*, 2018, p. 109.

48. Barker, B.S. et al. "Developing an elementary engineering education program through problem-based wearable technologies activities, " in *K-12 STEM Education: Breakthroughs in Research and Practice*, 2018, IGI Global. pp. 29–55.

49. Chen, J.A. et al. "Covid-19 and telepsychiatry: Early outpatient experiences and implications for the future," *General Hospital Psychiatry*, 66, 2020, 89–95.

50. Maheu, M.M. et al. *The mental health professional and the new technologies: A handbook for practice today*, 2004. Taylor & Francis.

51. Cosinuss. "Key study on Remote Patient Monitoring of Covid-19 patients," 2020, www.cosinuss.com/en/ (cited January 14, 2021).

52. Riede, J., *Sensorische Anfallsdetektion Bei Epilepsie*, 2019. Springer.

53. Rammohan, S.R., Niveditha, M.V. "Emerging technologies for mitigating the impact of the Covid-19 pandemic," *New Approaches in Commerce, Economics, Engineering, Humanities, Arts, Social Sciences and Management: Challenges and Opportunities*, p. 64.

54. Castro, E.I.B. et al. "Covid-19: Measures to prevent hospital contagion.What do urologists need to know?," *International braz j urol*, 46, 2020, 113–119.

55. PRO, A. Aranet PRO. 2020, https://aranet.com/product/wireless-iot-base-station-3/ (cited January 14, 2021).

56. Naik, B.N. et al. "Real-Time Smart Patient Monitoring and Assessment Amid Covid-19 Pandemic–an Alternative Approach to Remote Monitoring," *Journal of Medical Systems*, 44(7), 2020, 1–2.

57. Zhang, Y. et al. "Remote mobile health monitoring system based on smart phone and browser/server structure," *Journal of Healthcare Engineering*, 2015, 6.

58. Tabacof, L. et al. "Remote Patient Monitoring for Home Management of Coronavirus Disease 2019 in New York: A Cross-Sectional Observational Study," *Telemedicine and e-Health*, 2020.

59. Goyal, P. et al. "Clinical characteristics of Covid-19 in New York city," *New England Journal of Medicine*, 2020.

60. Khan, Y. et al. "Monitoring of vital signs with flexible and wearable medical devices," *Advanced Materials*, 28(22), 2016, 4373–4395.

61. Manta, C. et al. "An Evaluation of Biometric Monitoring Technologies for Vital Signs in the Era of COVID-19," *Clinical and Translational Science*, 13(6), 2020, 1034–1044.

62. Castaneda, D. et al. "A review on wearable photoplethysmography sensors and their potential future applications in health care," *International Journal of Biosensors & Bioelectronics*, 4(4), 2018, 195.

63. Baggish, A.L. et al. "Cardiovascular screening in college athletes with and without electrocardiography: a cross-sectional study," *Annals of Internal Medicine*, 152(5), 2010, 269–275.

64. Zhou, F. et al. "Clinical course and risk factors for mortality of adult inpatients with Covid-19 in Wuhan, China: a retrospective cohort study," *The Lancet*, 2020.

65. Reboussin, D.M. et al. "Systematic review for the 2017 ACC/AHA/AAPA/ABC/ACPM/AGS/APhA/ASH/ASPC/NMA/PCNA guideline for the prevention, detection, evaluation, and management of high blood pressure in adults: a report of the American College of Cardiology/American Heart Association Task Force on Clinical Practice Guidelines," *Journal of the American College of Cardiology*, 71(19), 2018, 2176–2198.

66. Muntner, P. et al. "Measurement of blood pressure in humans: a scientific statement from the American Heart Association," *Hypertension*, 73(5), 2019, e35–e66.

67. Del Sorbo, L. et al. "Mechanical ventilation in adults with acute respiratory distress syndrome. Summary of the experimental evidence for the clinical practice guideline," *Annals of the American Thoracic Society*, 14(Supplement 4), 2017, S261–S270.

68. Caputo, N.D., Strayer, R.J., Levitan, R. "Early Self-Proning in Awake, Non-intubated Patients in the Emergency Department: A Single ED's Experience During the COVID-19 Pandemic," *Academic Emergency Medicine*, 27(5), 2020, 375–378.

69. Marjanovic, N., Mimoz, O., Guenezan, J. "An easy and accurate respiratory rate monitor is necessary," *Journal of Clinical Monitoring and Computing*, 34(2), 2020, 221–222.

70. Kellett, J. et al. "Comparison of the heart and breathing rate of acutely ill medical patients recorded by nursing staff with those measured over 5 min by a piezoelectric belt and ECG monitor at the time of admission to hospital," *Resuscitation*, 82(11), 2011, 1381–1386.

71. Ahmed, M.U. "An intelligent healthcare service to monitor vital signs in daily life–A case study on health-IoT," *Int. J. Eng. Res. Appl.(IJERA)*, 7(3), 2017, 43–55.

72. Das, D. and Zhang, J. "Pandemic in a smart city: Singapore's Covid-19 management through technology & society," *Urban Geography*, 2020, 1–9.

73. Roy, D. et al. "Study of knowledge, attitude, anxiety & perceived mental healthcare need in Indian population during Covid-19 pandemic," *Asian Journal of Psychiatry*, 2020, 102083.

74. Otoom, M. et al. "An IoT-based framework for early identification and monitoring of Covid-19 cases," *Biomedical Signal Processing and Control*, 62, 2020, 102149.

75. Nausheen, F., Begum, S.H. "Healthcare IoT: benefits, vulnerabilities and solutions," in *2018 2nd International Conference on Inventive Systems and Control (ICISC)*, 2018. IEEE.

76. Blasco, J. et al. "A survey of wearable biometric recognition systems," *ACM Computing Surveys (CSUR)*, 49(3), 2016, 1–35.

11 Impact of IoT-Based Urban Agriculture on Healthcare

Smart Farms for Homes

Sanyam Arora, Luv Sethi, Shruti Agarwal, and Vimal Kumar
Department of Computer Science and Engineering
Meerut Institute of Engineering and Technology

CONTENTS

DOI: 10.1201/9781003146087-14

Covid-19 makes a strong case for urban farming. During the Covid lockdown, the food supply chain has been disrupted because of restrictions on logistics. So, to minimize the risk of infection, we are working on a solution to grow fruit and vegetables in concrete jungles. This method of growing food is known as "urban agriculture". With the help of emerging technologies such as the Internet of Things (IoT), we can make farming practices more systematic and well planned by reducing human intrusion through automation. This study aims to analyze and select the best method for urban agriculture with IoT and provide an overview of sensor data collection, automation, and the benefits of such technologies on healthcare. This chapter highlights the benefits of urban agriculture in healthcare by controlling the growing environment.

The high-tech methods used in urban farming ensures good yield and better health. With the use of IoT in our method, we can control and monitor the growth of plants and nutrient composition in soil. It also highlights the challenges expected to be faced while implementing these methods with traditional agricultural methods. And what would be the difference in the yield produced between both methods. The sensors are available for these applications, like crop growth status, irrigation, environment monitoring and soil nutrient parameters. This technology helps urban citizens to grow food organically in their space. We have analyzed various practices and methods used for urban agriculture and implemented the best methods. With the integration of IoT in it, we can completely automate the farming process and can create small farms in our homes to get healthy and organic food. The health of the community should be the prime goal of our food production system. The heavy use of chemicals, fertilizers, and pesticides harms our health and deteriorates the environment. So, the idea of urban agriculture is to grow organic food that will lead to better health and a better environment at a lower cost. The use of IoT with farming practices will make this process more efficient.

11.1   INTRODUCTION

Urban agriculture is the practice of growing food in or around urban areas. Urban agriculture is not only about growing food on rooftops. It involves turning any space within a city into a productive source of food. Backyards, parking lots and even the vacant space beside buildings can be converted into small urban farms [1]. The world is changing fast and, if we have to keep up with the pace of change, we need to change the way we produce food. The population is increasing, and the land for agriculture is decreasing. The food we eat deteriorates with harmful chemicals as producers have to produce food in large quantities in small spaces [2]. IoT is a technology that is set to change and improve agricultural practices. We can deploy IoT for smart farming (smart agriculture), but we the fundamental purpose remains the same:

After studying and analyzing various methods of urban agriculture like drip irrigation, vertical farming, hydroponics and some more, we have come up with our model of urban agriculture, which is IoT based [2,13,14]. We aim to provide nutrition-rich food without deteriorating the environment and health. It cannot be denied that the indiscriminate and excessive use of synthetic or inorganic fertilizers and pesticides have contaminated our food and environment. The toxic limit of fertilizer consumption/absorption may affect kidneys, lungs and is reported to cause cancer. The major effect is when toxic chemicals found in fertilizers are absorbed by plants and enter the food chain via vegetables and cereals. However, the largest health risk is contamination of groundwater, which is then used for drinking [9].

Emerging technologies like IoT are reforming and reshaping our conventional farming into smart farming. In this chapter, we will see how IoT enables us to increase the quality and quantity of food production. It also helps us reduce human labour, and human interventions using automation can add value to many aspects of farming. Using IoT we can intelligently control and analyze various factors like temperature, water, humidity and other parameters. These technologies are also helping urban gardeners to save time and resources. Wireless methods are used to collect data from different sensors at various nodes and send it through the wireless network. The collected data provides us with the required meaningful information about various environmental factors. This project shows various features such as smart decision making based on soil moisture, temperature, humidity, soil nutrients and other real-time data. For gathering the information of these parameters, sensors like soil moisture sensors, DHT11 sensors, level sensors, pH sensors and other customized sensors are used [6,8].

The highlights of the benefits of food grown by urban agriculture are also presented. It produces nutrition-rich and harmful chemical-free yields in good quantities. Urban agriculture helps us to build a healthy community.

11.2 URBAN AGRICULTURE

With the increase in population and the increase in demand for food, it has been a major problem to fulfil the demand for food. It causes an increase in the prices of vegetables. To overcome this issue, people have started practising urban agriculture. Urban agriculture is not just limited to growing food on rooftops. In addition, it consists of small and big landscapes in a city and turning them into a fruitful source of food. Backyards, roofs, balconies, parking lots and even the vacant space beside buildings can be converted into small-scale urban farms. Urban agriculture uses a very small amount of water to grow plants and vegetables, which also helps us to save money. The vegetables we grow are fresh and healthier than the vegetables available in the market. The main aim of urban farming is to grow vegetables for self-consumption [3]. As they are easier to grow, most people grow leafy vegetables in urban agriculture practices [1].

There are various urban agriculture practices: backyard gardens, greenhouses, rooftop gardens, green walls, vertical farms, aquaponics, hydroponics, agrobot, indoor farming.

11.2.1 BACKYARD GARDEN

In simple terms, a backyard garden refers to a home garden that can provide us with vegetables and fresh greens. Backyard gardening is a great method to address food security and health-related issues by producing fresh greens and vegetables grown near our home. It also promotes a healthy lifestyle.

11.2.2 GREENHOUSES

Greenhouses facilitate high tech production of vegetables, fruits, edible greens and flowers. The roofs of greenhouses are made up of transparent material like glass or plastic sheets. The temperature inside becomes warmer because sunlight is trapped inside by the transparent roof. It enables the grower to produce vegetables or other edible greens all-round the year. In a greenhouse, we can optimize a plant's growth by controlling many factors like heating, cooling, humidity [3]. Different types of greenhouses are available based on their technical specifications.

11.2.3 ROOFTOP GARDENS

Rooftop gardens are very popular among urban gardeners. The technique of cultivating food on the rooftop of buildings is known as rooftop farming. Rooftop gardens can be helpful to grow our food. We can use various methods like vertical farming on our rooftops. The concept of rooftop farming can contribute to food security in urban areas.

11.2.4 GREEN WALL

A green wall is a vertical greening typology, where a vertical built structure is covered by vegetation. Green walls are different from vertical farms. In green walls, the plants are grown on the surface or structure of the wall, whereas in vertical farms, the plants are grown on different levels. Apart from producing edible greens, green walls have additional benefits as they also reduce the temperature of buildings [21].

11.2.5 VERTICAL FARMS

Vertical farming is a method of urban farming used to produce food vertically in layers [5]. Vertical farming is a popular method of urban agriculture nowadays. As the population is increasing, land acquisition by humans is increasing. So, the demand for food also increases, but the land for growing plants and food decreases [6]. To overcome this situation, this urban farming method helps to grow a large number of plants and food in less area. Conventional farming uses up to 65–70% of available freshwater; so, water scarcity has increased. This method of urban agriculture uses up to 95% less water than conventional farming, which also helps us to save water. This method of urban farming grows the plants with the help of natural resources rather than fossils. The basic and the most important advantage of vertical farming is that we can grow plants and food anywhere and anytime [4]. This popular method has been acquired by many countries (United States, Japan, Sweden, Singapore, and the Netherlands). It may become the most important sector of the food industry in future as it can grow more food in less area [4].

11.2.6 AQUAPONICS

Aquaponics is a type of agricultural practice that includes raising fish and other aquatic animals in tanks with soilless plant culture. In simple terms, we can say that aquaponics is a combination of hydroponics and aquaculture.

Hydroponics refers to growing plants in water, and aquaculture refers to raising fish in tanks, which helps provide nutrients to the water. Hence an ecosystem is established: plants help clean the water for the fish, and fish excrete works as a natural fertilizer for the plants. The major benefit of this method is that we do not need to add additional fertilizers. The fish waste acts as fertilizer, which plays a vital role in the plant's growth. The waste also contains beneficial bacteria and microbes that accumulate in the confined area between the plant roots present in the ecosystem and converts the leftovers from fish into material that plants can use for their growth.

We can achieve two goals simultaneously using aquaponics: the first is raising fish and the second is producing fresh vegetables [20].

11.2.7 HYDROPONICS

Hydroponics (Figure 11.1) is a technique for growing plants in water without soil. Growing plants in soil with less culture or hydroponics is an ancient technique (ancient examples of hydroponics include the Hanging Gardens of Babylon and the Floating Gardens of China). According to some hydroponic farmers, the yields they get are much more than those from conventional methods. In hydroponically grown plants, the roots have emerged into nutrient-rich solutions as they can directly absorb required nutrients from the solution. The plants commonly grown hydroponically on inert media include lettuces, spinach, tomatoes, strawberries, peppers, cucumbers and many more.

There are many advantages of hydroponics over conventional farming. It is observed that plants grow faster hydroponically as compared to soil-based farming. This is because the roots of the plants get more oxygen, which helps them to absorb nutrition faster. The plant does not need to find nutrition from the soil. The water-based nutrient solution contains all the elements plants normally would get from the soil for healthy growth. Hydroponically grown plants are healthier as they are less prone to bug infestations, fungus, and disease [2].

Different types of hydroponic systems are available. Many factors are considered while selecting a hydroponic system: the type of plant being grown, available space, cost and many more.

Hydroponic systems can be classified as active or passive. In an active hydroponic system, the nutrient solution steadily moves using a pump. In contrast, the nutrient solution is absorbed by the growing medium using capillary action in a passive hydroponic system. They can also be classified as recovery or non-recovery systems. In

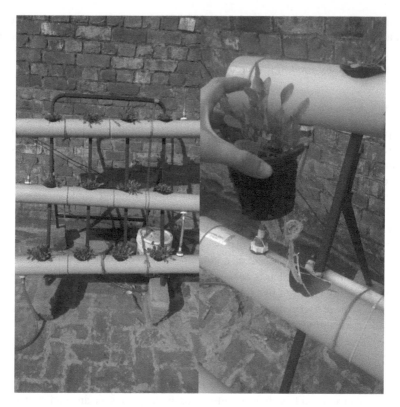

FIGURE 11.1   Our experimental hydroponic setup.

a recovery system, the nutrient solution is reused or recirculated, whereas in non-recovery, the nutrient solution is not reused or recirculated [3].

Some of the widely used hydroponic systems are the wick system, deep water culture (DWC), ebb and flow, the drip system, nutrient film technology (NFT) and aeroponic systems [2].

11.2.7.1   Wick System

The wick system (Figure 11.2) is one of the simplest methods of hydroponics. It is a passive hydroponic system. It does not require any pump. The plants are placed in a growing medium like cocopeat, vermiculite with a wick. Wick is any absorbent material that runs from the plant into a reservoir. The nutrients solution is stored in the reservoir, and it is supplied into the root of the plant by capillary action.

Advantages

The wick system is easy to install and maintain. It is inexpensive.

Disadvantages

This system is not efficient to supply a lot of nutrition to plants. Therefore, it works well only for small herbs and plants.

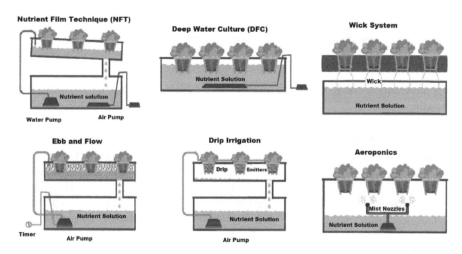

FIGURE 11.2 Types of hydroponics.

11.2.7.2 Ebb and Flow

Ebb and flow (Figure 11.2) is an active and recovery kind of hydroponic system. It is also known as the flood and drain system. This method uses a submersible pump in the reservoir, and the plants are placed in a tray. It works on a simple flood and drain concept. The reservoir contains the nutrient solution and the pump. The nutrient solution is pumped up to the upper tray when power is on and is supplied to the plant's roots. The duration in which the pump is on is called a flood cycle. When the water reaches a set level, the nutrient solution is allowed to overflow. The process is called the flood cycle. The nutrient solution drains back down into the reservoir using the pump. The pump remains active during the flood cycle as well.

Advantages

It is comparatively low maintenance and an effective system. It provides nutrition to plants in abundance.

Disadvantages

Many risks are involved using this system. When the nutrient solution is drained back into the nutrient reservoir from the growth tray, the solution changes dramatically, which can damage the plants.

11.2.7.3 Deep Water Culture

Deep water culture (Figure 11.2) is an active type of hydroponic growing method in which the roots of the plants are sustained in a well-oxygenated and nutrition-rich solution of water 24/7.

A reservoir is filled with water, and required nutrients are added. Also, the pH of the solution is maintained. In this method, an air pump is connected to an air-stone which is placed inside the reservoir. Plants are placed in net pots above the nutrient solution such that plants emerge from their roots and absorb nutrients from the solution.

Advantages

It is a widely used method. It requires low maintenance.

Disadvantages

It is important to check on pH and nutrition level; otherwise, it may hinder the plant's growth.

11.2.7.4 Drip System

An active type of hydroponic system is well known as the drip system (Figure 11.2). The nutrient solution is pumped to the base of the plants through the tube, and the tube contains holes that allow the nutrient solution to reach the plants. The nutrient solution passed to the plants is placed below the grow bed, as in the ebb and flow technique.

Advantages

It can provide nutrition to the plant efficiently.

Disadvantages

The main problem is that the nutrients and pH of the solution change when water is recirculated.

11.2.7.5 Nutrition Film Technique

An active and recovery kind of hydroponic technique is also known as the nutrient film technique (Figure 11.2). This system contains a submersible pump, which is the part of the reservoir that pumps the nutrient solution into a grow tube. The roots of the plant are submerged in the grow tray. The nutrient solution circulates from the roots (in the tube) to the reservoir, so the grow-tube is placed slightly downwards.

Advantages

It is an efficient technique for large-scale production.

Disadvantages

Power supply issues can destroy the plant.

11.2.7.6 Aeroponic System

Aeroponics (Figure 11.2) is a system in which plants are suspended in the air to grow. A tank is placed below the plants, along with a water pump. Nozzles are attached to that pump; they sprinkle water when the pressure increases and reaches a certain limit.

Advantages

It is an efficient method of growing plants in a limited space using less material.

Disadvantages

This system is expensive. It requires technical knowledge for running and maintaining the system. Unbalanced nutrients can kill the plant.

11.3 INTERNET OF THINGS

IoT is a machine-to-machine network embedded in devices like microcontrollers or microprocessors that processes data from sensors or command actuators. These devices can be ordinary household appliances or industrial machines that communicate through wireless networks and work without any human interaction [11,13]. IoT devices are usually low-power, limited processing capacity, have small memory, are cheaper in cost, and have resource-constrained devices [15]. Communication for IoT devices is done by applying cloud-based publishing and subscribing methods. Publishing and subscribing methods interact by a message from the device to device, based on specified topics. Components that generate messages are known as publishers, while those that receive messages are known as subscribers. It means a broker acting as an intermediate in between makes communication between publisher and subscriber. They are not aware of the existence of each other. They only communicate by having a broker in between. A broker acts as a receiver and filters the message, then forwards it to subscribers concerning node-topic. Brokers are identified with their port number and IP address. A node can act as a publisher or a subscriber with the intermediate broker and interchange data from other nodes. The publisher sends a message with a node topic, which the broker then reviews to analyze the subscriber of that message according to the specified topic. There are various protocols of communication of IoT devices like Constrained Application Protocol (CoAP), Message Queuing Telemetry Transport (MQTT), Advanced Message Queuing Protocol (AMQP) and Lightweight M2M (LwM2M). Among these MQTT is the most used protocol for consumer IoT devices. MQTT is an IoT or M2M protocol that uses publishing and subscribing methods to communicate among different nodes, shown in (Figure 11.3).

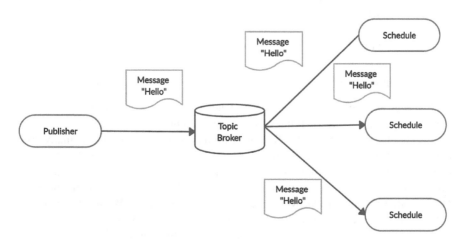

FIGURE 11.3 Working of MQTT.

MQTT is a lightweight protocol designed for low power devices like embedded systems and mobile devices, which comprise limited resources. MQTT works great on low bandwidth, high-latency and unreliable networks. MQTT ensures the delivery of messages between nodes and servers. It is a message-based information transfer protocol. It is ideally suitable for IoT devices having limited capabilities and resources. MQTT connection involves two agents: MQTT broker and MQTT clients. A device that is connected to the network and exchanges messages through MQTT is called an MQTT client, which can either be a subscriber or publisher. Publishers publish information in the form of messages and subscriber requests for the messages. MQTT broker is a device or program that interconnects the MQTT clients. Devices like microcontrollers or microprocessors that are connected to various sensors or actuators are typically the MQTT clients. When a client has to send a message to the node, it forwards the data to the MQTT broker. The MQTT broker is then responsible for organizing and filtering the data. All the data published by clients (MQTT nodes) are forwarded to other nodes subscribed to it (subscriber nodes). This protocol simplifies the process of communication by abstracting all the methodology into a broker. MQTT protocol acts as a middleware to connect clients. Still, to be able to communicate with each other, this middleware requires a formatting language. There are many languages that support this task like node.js, Lua, Python, JSON and more. Still, JSON is widely used to exchange information [16]. The data is sent or received using the publish and subscribe methods. There can be various devices like cellphones or computers, which could act as an intermediate to send or receive data.

This is an example JSON format:

{"setup":{"sensors":{"ph":7.24,"temp":28.86,"hm":96,"c":10},
"actuator":{"pM1":120,"pM2":200,"pM3":96," relay":1}}

In the given data, we described the complete setup containing two sub-nodes: the sensor node and actuator node. The sensor node is further communicated with sensors connected to the node, in our case, pH, temperature, humidity and soil moisture. The actuator nodes are connected to various actuators connected with the node, relays and peristaltic pumps.

11.3.1 Methodology

With the growth in urbanization, fewer land spaces are available in metropolitan areas. Due to this, the availability of fresh and organic food becomes less, and these are also being sold in the market for a very high cost. To solve this issue, many urban agriculture practices are now being practised by people in urban areas. Most of these practices have been described in this chapter. Not all these practices are easy to be implemented by a novice, so we have focused on the pros of various methods and implemented a solution that would be feasible in the budget. We tried to automate most of the process, which would require lesser or no manpower.

The experimental setup platform is made after studying the structure of indoor vertical farming, hydroponics like nutrient film technology, aeroponics, rooftop gardening and greenhouse. The structure is built with four PVC tubes attached on a metal stand to make it vertical in position and with which we could grow more vegetation in less space. Each tube comprises several netted pots filled with cocopeat, perlite and clay pebbles. These were sown in the water overnight and then used. Netted pots used in the experimental setup were 3.5 inches in diameter and are 3 inches in height. Soil moisture sensors and water level sensors have been used to make an analysis. Soil moisture sensors are placed inside the pots. PVC tubes are connected with the nutrient pump, which is kept in a covered bucket, and all the pipes are connected to make water flow in it. The nutrient bucket is filled with water, a small amount of organic N, P, K solution available on the market and a small seaweed solution. We have focused on the growth of spinach, monitoring its full growth, and finding out the chemical composition required to grow spinach. The overall process of controlling and monitoring our planting setup is shown (Figure 11.4). According to this figure, with the availability of a network, the smart farming system acts as both subscriber and a publisher and connects to the MQTT broker. The user from his device can publish to the broker to get the sensors' information or control the actuator (pump). The water valve and water pump will be turned on, and the user can also control the flow of water from his device when the user presses the 'on' button in the web browser. In our case, a soil moisture sensor detects the humidity of the soil, a DHT11 sensor is used to determine the temperature and humidity of the

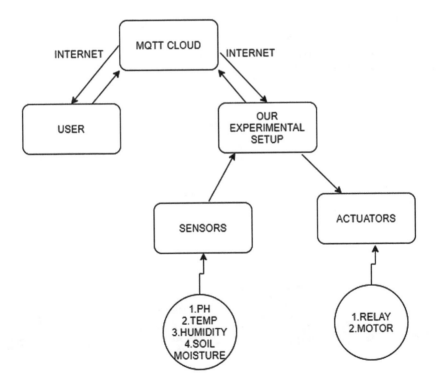

FIGURE 11.4 Flowchart of our experimental setup.

environment, a pH sensor is connected in the water flow bucket to maintain the pH in water, and all the nutrients are connected with a peristaltic pump to control the nutrient supplied in water.

11.3.2 COMPONENTS USED

- ESP32
- Soil moisture
- pH sensor
- Dht11
- Peristaltic pump
- Relays
- Motor driver

11.3.2.1 ESP 32

ESP 32 (Figure 11.5) is integrated with dual-mode Bluetooth and Wi-Fi in it. ESP 32 is a low power, low-cost system in a chip [7]. It is robust and capable of working from −40C to +125C [6]. ESP 32 can dynamically remove the imperfections in the external circuit and even adapt to the changes that have occurred in the external conditions.

11.3.2.2 Soil Moisture Sensor

Soil moisture (Figure 11.5) sensor measures both air and water temperature in the soil. While using the soil moisture sensor, relative humidity becomes an important factor to study. The relative humidity is the ratio of air to the highest amount of moisture at a particular temperature [6].

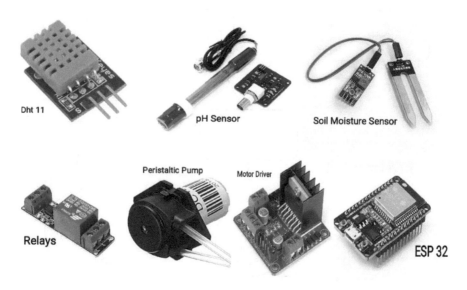

FIGURE 11.5 Components used.

11.3.2.3   Dht 11

Dht 11(Figure 11.5) is a combined module that can sense humidity and temperature, giving a digital output. Dht11 gives us very precise values of humidity and temperature. Dht11 works on single-wire communication. It is an NTC type temperature measurement sensor with an 8-bit microcontroller built in [8].

11.3.2.4   P.H. Sensor

The H+ ions present in the water helps us to measure the pH of water. The more H+ ions in the solution, the more is the acidic character of the solution, and the less is the H+ ions in the solution, the more is the alkaline character of the solution. The sensor (Figure 11.5) can measure the pH in all ionic strength conditions. The accuracy of the pH sensor is ± 0.1 unit, and it ranges from 0 to 14 units and gives the resolution of 0.01 unit [9].

11.3.2.5   Peristaltic Pump

This is a type of displacement pump that can pump a variety of fluids. It comprises certain gears like structures that rotate and pressurize the water inside the flexible tube and flow.

11.3.2.6   Relays

A relay (Figure 11.5) is electrically operated, and it works as a switch. Relays are used for circuits with low power signals or where two or more circuits need to be controlled by a single signal. When the microcontroller generates the output, the relay turns on. NPN transistors are used in the relays [17].

11.3.2.7   Motor Driver

A motor driver (Figure 11.5) is used to control and give power to a motor. The microcontroller sends the signal to the motor driver, and the motor driver performs the function as a switch. The switch then gives the required voltage to the motors to perform the function. A motor driver can control two motors at a time. It has a capacity of 2 amperes per channel and can give output up to 45 volts [10].

11.4   IMPACT ON HEALTHCARE AND BENEFITS

Urban agriculture ensures the availability of fresh food. The dependence on processed food is reduced with the food grown by urban agriculture, moving towards a healthy society and reducing the risk of lifestyle diseases. With our experimental setup, we obtained a high yield of spinach (Figure 11.6) compared to the land of the same size, which was grown without any additional harmful chemicals. Urban agriculture farms are designed to minimize water consumption and eliminate the use of harmful chemicals, which eliminates toxicity in food and the use of water. In today's generation of fast food and packed food, we lack nutrition-rich and fibrous food. As a result, we face numerous health issues such as blood pressure, obesity, diabetes. These instant options like packed food may be faster, but they are not good for health as they are loaded with preservatives and artificial flavours. Urban agriculture enables us to grow our own healthy and nutritious food like fruits, vegetables, and herbs. The greens grown are rich in nutrients and have beneficial vitamins. Most urban farmers make sure that the greens grown are free from harmful pesticides and fertilizers and use good soil, water, fertilizer. IT helps us to get better quality and quantity of food. Light can be bent or refracted by the nutrients present in the liquid and can be measured using a refractometer. This can be used in measuring the nutritional values in liquids.

We have compared our grown spinach (Figure 11.6) with those available in the market. There are not many differences in the shape and size, except the one grown in our home is fresher and cleaner than that bought from the market. And it is also completely free from any harmful chemicals, insecticides and pesticides, and so is good for healthcare. Our setup is highly flexible and can be optimized to grow medicinal plants [18].

11.5 CONCLUSION

IoT-based urban agriculture focuses on efficient and smarter farming practices for producing healthy yields. In this chapter, we have observed various methods for growing

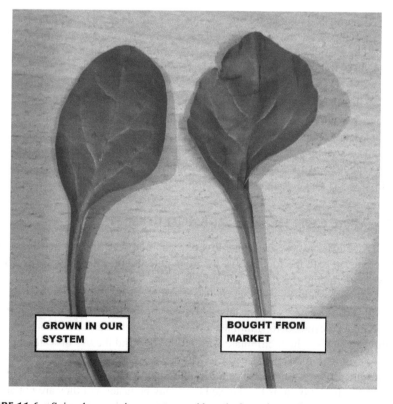

FIGURE 11.6   Spinach grown in our setup and bought from the market.

crops in urban areas and have practised our methods of growing crops by combining various methods. And the results showed that we could get a better yield of vegetables from our method in a much smaller area. We have also shown the healthcare benefits and also what parameters our experiment can control. For this purpose, we have used IoT. We have easily automated technology using various sensors and actuators and made it more efficient and beneficial for human healthcare. Plants grown using these methods are more fresh and good for healthcare as this method does not use any harmful chemicals and fertilizers.

Furthermore, a deeper insight into various methodologies and their advantages and disadvantages has been provided. In addition, mostly used IoT methodologies have been explored, together with use cases concerning agriculture applications. A summary of methods to grow plants through urban agriculture methods has been listed to guide readers. Based on this, it can be concluded that even in very small areas far from big farms, plants can grow plants without the need for human interaction.

REFERENCES

1. Orsini, F., Kahane, R., Nono-Womdim, R. et al. "Urban agriculture in the developing world: a review," *Agronomy for Sustainable Development*, 33, 2013, 695–720.
2. Pawar, I.S., Tembe, S., Acharekar, R., Khan, S., Yadav, S., "Design of an IoT enabled Automated Hydroponics system using NodeMCU and Blynk," *2019 IEEE 5th International Conference for Convergence in Technology (I2CT)*, 2019.
3. Ayaz, M., Ammad, M., Sharif-Uddin, Z., Mansour, A., Aggoune, E.-H.M., "Internet-of-Things (IoT)-Based Smart Agriculture: Toward Making the Fields Talk," in *IEEE Access*, 7, 2019, 129551–129583.
4. Kalantari, Fatemeh, Mohd Tahir, Osman, Lahijani, Ahmad Mahmoudi, Kalantari, Shahaboddin. "A review of vertical farming technology: a guide for implementation of building integrated agriculture in cities," *Advanced Engineering Forum*, 24, 2017, 76–91.
5. Chowdhury, Muhammad E.H., Khandakar, Amith, Ahmed, Saba, Al-Khuzaei, Fatima, Hamdalla, Jalaa, Haque, Fahmida, Reaz, Mamun B.I., Al Shafei, Ahmed, Al-Emadi, Nasser. "Design, Construction and Testing of IoT Based Automated Indoor Vertical Hydroponics Farming Test-Bed in Qatar," *Sensors* 20(19), 2020.
6. Raza, Saleem, Faheem, Muhammad, Günes, Mesut. "Industrial wireless sensor and actuator networks in industry 4.0: Exploring requirements, protocols, and challenges-A MAC survey," *International Journal of Communication Systems*, 32, 2019.
7. Kodali, R.K., Valdas, A., "MQTT Based Monitoring System for Urban Farmers Using ESP32 and Raspberry Pi," *2018 Second International Conference on Green Computing and Internet of Things (ICGCIoT)*, 2018.
8. Sharmila, F. Margret, Suryaganesh, P., Abishek, M., Benny, U., "Iot Based Smart Window using Sensor Dht11," *2019 5th International Conference on Advanced Computing & Communication Systems (ICACCS)*, 2019.
9. Pujar, P.M., Kenchannavar, H.H., Kulkarni, R.M., Kulkarni, U.P., "Real-time water quality monitoring through Internet of Things and ANOVA-based analysis: a case study on river Krishna", 10(1), 2019.
10. Tir, Z., Malik, O., Hamida, M.A., Cherif, H., Bekakra, Y., Kadrine, A., "Implementation of a fuzzy logic speed controller for a permanent magnet dc motor using a low-cost Arduino platform," *2017 5th International Conference on Electrical Engineering – Boumerdes (ICEE-B)*, 2017.

11. Suresh, K., Kumar, G.V., "Integrated Cloud Internet of Things for Realtime Applications," *2020 Fourth International Conference on I-SMAC (IoT in Social, Mobile, Analytics and Cloud) (I-SMAC)*, 2020.

12. Buyya, Rajkumar, Marusic, Slaven, Palaniswami, Marimuthu, "Internet of Things (IoT): A vision, architectural elements, and future directions," *Future Generation Computer Systems*, 29(7), 2013.

13. Yadav, E.P., Mittal, E.A., Yadav, H., "IoT: Challenges and Issues in Indian Perspective," *2018 3rd International Conference On Internet of Things: Smart Innovation and Usages (IoT-SIU)*, 2018.

14. Razzaque, Mohammad Abdur, Milojevic, Marija, Palade, Andrei, Clarke, Siobhán. "Middleware for Internet of Things: A Survey," *IEEE Internet of Things Journal*, 3, 2015, 70–95.

15. Asghar, M.H., Mohammadzadeh, N. "Design and simulation of energy efficiency in node based on MQTT protocol in Internet of Things," *2015 International Conference on Green Computing and Internet of Things (ICGCIoT)*, 2015.

16. Kalliatakis, Grigorios, Stergiou, Alexandros, Vidakis, Nikolaos. "Conceiving Human Interaction by Visualizing Depth Data of Head Pose Changes and Emotion Recognition via Facial Expressions," *Computers*, 6(3), 2017, 25.

17. Laluma, R.H., Giantara, R., Sugiarto, B., Gunawan, Siregar, C.A., Risnanto, S., "Automation System of Water Treatment Plant using Raspberry Pi.3 Model B+ Based on Internet of Things (IoT)," *2019 IEEE 13th International Conference on Telecommunication Systems, Services, and Applications (TSSA)*, 2019.

18. Hossain Chowdhury, Mohammad Shaheed, Koike, Masao, Muhammed, Nur, Halim, Md. Abdul, Saha, Narayan, Kobayashi, Hajime, "Use of plants in healthcare: a traditional ethno-medicinal practice in rural areas of southeastern Bangladesh," *International Journal of Biodiversity Science & Management*, 5(1), 2009, 41–51,

19. "Figure Wick System," *Basic Hydroponic Systems and How They Work*, www.simplyhydro.com/system/.

20. "Figure types of Hydroponics," *Types of Hydroponics*: www.nosoilsolutions.com/6-different-types-hydroponic-systems/.

21. "Aquaponics," *What is Aquaponics*, https://aquaponics.com/aquaponics-in-schools/aquaponics-information/.

12 Identification of Heavy Drinking by Using IoT Devices and Artificial Intelligence

Karan Gupta and Ritin Behl
Department of Information Technology
ABES Engineering College

Luv Dhamija
Department of Computer Science and Engineering
ABES Engineering College

CONTENTS

Many people worldwide succumb to death due to the consumption of alcohol in large quantities. These circumstances are more likely to happen when an individual is drinking at a public place as they become unconscious and lose control over themselves, eventually resulting in fatal accidents. To overcome this problem, several wearable devices have been introduced that can detect the amount of alcohol present inside a person's body and alert the person if he goes beyond a certain limit. But these devices are very costly, and hence not every individual can afford them.

DOI: 10.1201/9781003146087-15

203

To find other alternatives, we saw that it is possible to apply the Internet of Things (IoT) and machine learning to classify the state of a person using their smartphone's sensor data. The main objective of this chapter is to detect whether a specific user has consumed alcohol over a permissible limit or not by using data retrieved from phone sensors, as these sensors can recognise the user's movements due to the after-effects of heavy drinking. Different kinds of research develop unique inferences about this data gathered from the sensors of the smartphones; however, they do not make general use of user's information. Since the data generated is time-dependent, we try to build various hybrid long short term memory (LSTM) models and compare the accuracy of each one with the existing predictive models proposed by other researchers. These models are more effective in assigning appropriate weights to every unit in a given time frame, but they can learn to identify an important input stored in the hidden states. Finally, the model can classify the person's behaviour based on the information gathered throughout the drinking episode.

12.1   INTRODUCTION

Deciding whether to consume alcohol or not is a personal choice, but it can prove to be fatal when done carelessly. If individuals are involved in a binge-drinking episode and consume alcohol over a specified limit, they tend to lose control over their senses. Excessive drinking is most common in college students as they are typically more involved in heavy drinking episodes. According to the 2018 NSDUH, approximately 861,000 people (about 2.3%) ages 12–20 (2.6% of males and 1.9% of females) reported heavy alcohol use in the past month [1][2]. Heavy alcohol consumption leads to various health issues, but it has many other indirect negative consequences such as motor accidents [3], assaulting another person, rapes [4], and unintentional injuries. Several preventive measures and proposals have been put forward throughout the years to spread awareness to students regarding the consequences of excessive alcohol consumption [5]. Different kinds of interventions such as education programmes [6], motivational feedback [7], and social media campaigns [8] have been conducted. Blood alcohol concentration (BAC) measurement is an important feature to determine the sobriety of a person. There are various methods to estimate BAC [9]. However, most of them are impractical to use in a real-time scenario. Electronic intervention approaches using sensors have become more popular and reliable as they can potentially avoid risks related to excessive alcohol consumption [10]. Vehicle-based sensors could be feasible to prevent car accidents due to alcohol impairment [11].

12.2   USING IOT DEVICES AND ARTIFICIAL INTELLIGENCE

There is an essential need to develop non-invasive and inconspicuous BAC monitoring to confront this situation. Meanwhile, about 1% of alcohol consumed discharges by sweat [12]; noticing alcohol released from the skin through a means known as transdermal alcohol detection (TAC) and deriving BAC values from these measures is a hopeful way to go about in this research. There are two instruments for measuring TAC sensors that are widely available. i.e., SCRAM™ and WrisTAS™, which are based on electrochemical transducers. The SCRAM™ is used in law-enforcement areas, whereas the WrisTAS™ for research purposes. Several studies have been directed to estimate both devices' performance. However, the large structure of the two devices means that they are not suitable to be worn for casual purposes. TAC sensors can detect the alcohol concentration in a person's body by analysing the alcohol that perspires through the skin [13]. TAC sensors are useful for remote monitoring, but these devices are expensive and require the person to wear it all the time, even though it is heavy. Nowadays, many smartphone applications have been introduced to deliver just-in-time interventions to the user by analysing the input data [14, 15]. These applications require the user to input some real-time data into the application. However, if this intervention has to be done frequently, it can be irritating for the person, and hence it cannot be of any help. This stipulates the need for a more advanced system that can accurately measure the person's current state and deliver a message only if there is a risk associated with further drinking. To develop a more convenient model for detecting a person's sobriety, we could use electronic sensors embedded in smartphones. Sensors such as accelerometers and gyroscopes can help identify position and orientation at a given point in time.

Data gathered from these sensors could help in identifying the behaviour of a person while walking. By identifying the walking behaviour, one could generalise whether a person has drunk over a certain limit or not. This approach is more advantageous than the ones mentioned previously. The user does not need to input any data from their end. The cost is also very low since accelerometers are readily available in most smartphone nowadays. The accelerometer data consists of acceleration in three-dimensions i.e., x, y, and z. All of these axes collectively determine the physical movement of a person, as described in Figure 12.1.

In our research, we use deep learning approaches and built several hybrid LSTM models that could be applied to this dataset since it is a time-series dataset. The advantage of using LSTM over other predictive machine learning models is that they do not require extra information about the data. In contrast, it is required to obtain the most relevant features for machine learning predictive models to improve the model's accuracy. Our study used variants of the LSTM networks and then compared their performances with each other. The ConvLSTM model was given the best accuracy as it performs convolution operations on input data and then applies the LSTM layers for sequence analysis.

The main concern here is to handle the problem of over-drinking and its attendant health risks, long term as well as short term. A solution is possible by integrating IoT with artificial intelligence. It is specifically advantageous for teenagers and adults who drink more than their capacity, unknowingly putting their lives at risk. The readings from IoT sensor devices such as MQ-3, an alcohol level detector by breath and the calculations done by the machine learning model provides a better way of assessing this problem with minimum human effort, giving people's health a priority.

12.2.1 Dataset

The data used for the research is available on the UCI Machine Learning Repository and was collected in 2017 in a study [16]. The dataset contains 13 different participants,

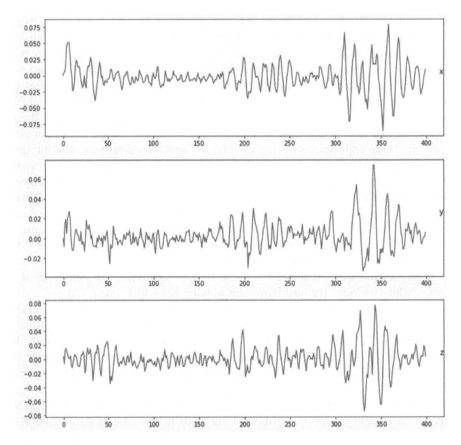

FIGURE 12.1   Plot of acceleration in each axis.

out of which 11 participants were using iPhones, and two were using Android phones. Participants were made to wear the SCRAM sensors to keep track of TAC values at different timestamps. Besides that, the dataset also contains values of accelerometer data in the x, y, and z axes with corresponding time stamps. The TAC values were calculated every half hour, and the acceleration data consists of values with a frequency of 40Hz per second.

12.2.2   DATA PRE-PROCESSING

All the data was dropped for which there were missing values of accelerometer data or TAC values. Only data that consisted of both values were taken into account. Since the TAC values were measured every half hour, all those values were mapped with the accelerometer data present in between that interval. After merging all the data, the TAC values were converted into two classes using a threshold of 0.8. Above the threshold were classified as "intoxicated", and below the threshold were "sober". Since every participant had different behaviour throughout the drinking episode,

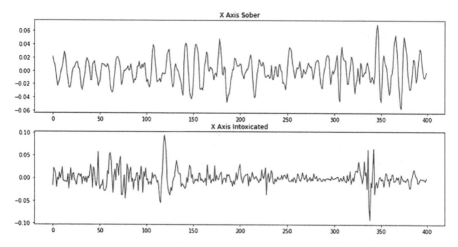

FIGURE 12.2   Plot of sober and intoxicated values on each axis.

some were more drunk than others, and some were less. In the final model, few more participant data were eliminated because it could not train the model. Figure 15.2 shows the comparison between a sober and intoxicated state in all three dimensions.

12.2.3   METHODOLOGY

This research uses different LSTM models to perform accurate predictions on the given data as this is a time-series problem [17, 18]. LSTM networks are a special kind of recurrent neural network (RNN), which can acquire long-term dependence [19]. It is also described as a black box that is mainly used as a basic cell except that it can perform more robustly, has faster training coverage, and has the feature to detect long-term dependencies present in the data. It mainly implements an optimised approach when working with the help of a GPU. LSTM has the property to recognise an important input stored in the long-term state, pressure it for as long as it requires and extract it whether necessary [20]. These mainly consist of three gates:

- Forget Gate(f_t): It generally controls which portion of the long-term state should be removed
- Input Gate(i_t): It generally controls which portion of (g_t) should be added to the long-term state.
- Output Gate(o_t): It generally controls which portion of the long-term state should be taken as input and output at the particular time [21,22].

Since every individual has their gait behaviour and has a different capacity for drinking [20], so it is better to fit the model to every participant and then see how well the model performs rather than generalising it for the whole sample. In our final stage, we used data of only eight participants because data of other participants were not ideal for training the model due to the low availability of intoxicated acceleration data for some participants and sober data for other participants.

12.2.4 Deep LSTM

A deep LSTM model is a kind of architecture that consists of several layers of LSTM that are stacked with each other. The output of one layer is passed as an input to the other, which eventually enhances the final performance of the model. These deep LSTM networks have the capability for higher representations of the sequence data [23]. To overcome overfitting so that our model performs well on the test data, we have used the L2 regularise [24, 25]. It could be used as a trade-off between the generalisation of the model and its complexity. We set the loss coefficient as 0.0015. In addition to this, we used the adaptive movement estimation, i.e. the Adam optimiser, for faster convergence and avoiding the problem of getting stuck at local minima. Finally, the model was implemented in python 3.6 using TensorFlow 1.15, which was solely run on a 4GB NVIDIA GeForce GTX 1050Ti GPU. The network consisted of two fully connected layers and three LSTM layers that are stacked together. For every sample of data, there were 200 rows of data, which means a window of five seconds as the frequency is 40 Hz with 100-time steps, so there was a 50% overlapping of the data.

Furthermore, for each LSTM layer, there were 40 hidden units present. The model was trained with 20 epochs. It took around one hour to train the model for every participant and eight hours in total for the whole model. After fitting the model, it was found out that the maximum accuracy for one of the participants came out at 88.44 %, and the minimum accuracy came out at 81.09%. This accuracy is better than the one obtained from conventional machine learning algorithms.

12.2.5 Bi-Directional LSTM

The bidirectional LSTMs model shown in Figure 12.3 is an extension over the traditional LSTM architecture. A basic LSTM keeps only the former information for prediction. As the name suggests, bidirectional LSTMs works in two directions

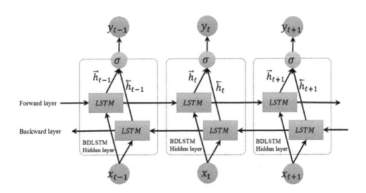

FIGURE 12.3 Representation of the bidirectional LSTM model.

rather than one to consider former and future information. Since they can work in two directions, they can predict more accurately on sequence classification problems. A bidirectional LSTM will read the input sequence in different manners [26, 27]. Firstly, it will read the input sequence as it is. Secondly, it will read the input sequence in a reversed manner. So it has a forward direction state, and a backward direction state, both of them are together responsible for the output [28, 29, 30].

Our experiment used an LSTM layer with 20 hidden units and wrapped it inside the bidirectional layer. As a result, the next layer of the model will receive 20 units of forwarding sequence and 20 units of backward sequence, 40 units. We used Adam optimiser for convergence as we did in the case of deep LSTM. It took a total of five hours to train and validate the model on all eight participants.

It was observed that bidirectional LSTM increased the accuracy with a small value for six of the participants. However, the accuracy decreased for two participants. It is, however, more efficient than traditional machine learning algorithms.

12.2.6 ConvLSTM

ConvLSTM, represented in Figure 12.4, is a further extension of the LSTM that can perform feature extraction before passing the data to the LSTM [31]. Convolution can be defined as an operation that slides one function on another and, finally, it calculates the integral of their pointwise multiplication. When this operation is implemented as a basic method to build a neural network, it is described as a convolution neural network. This network is a non-linear activation function applied to the results of convolutional operation, and then a full connection layer is used after the pooling operation for classification. ConvLSTM is a type of LSTM that consists of a convolution operation inside the LSTM cell. Both the models are the types of RNN, which can learn

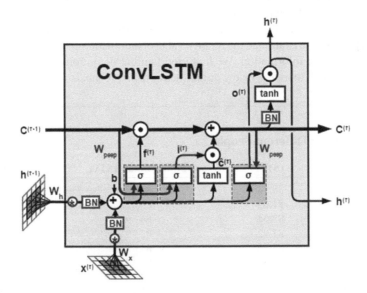

FIGURE 12.4 Representation of the ConvLSTM.

long-term dependencies. It changes the matrix multiplication with the convolution operation at every gate of the LSTM cell. Due to this, it seizes the hidden spatial features by this operation in multidimensional data [32, 33].

In the experiment, each sample had a window of five seconds with 200-time steps. There was a 50% overlapping by stepping with 100-time steps at every sample. There were 64 filters in the ConvLSTM layer. The activation function used for the model was rectified linear unit [34]. After that, the output was flattened into a single dimension vector. Finally, a softmax activation function was applied to perform classification for the two classes. The model was fit for 20 epochs, and the binary cross-entropy function was used for calculating the loss in the training process. The model took ten hours for the training.

12.3   RESULTS

After trying different LSTM models, we found that the ConvLSTM model performed better than bidirectional LSTM and deep LSTM. Table 12.1 shows the comparison between the three models in terms of their accuracy, with its corresponding participant ID. It was useful for classifying between intoxicated and sober states. This model can be used for smartphone applications for JITAIs (just in time interventions). The performance of each classifier is represented in Figure 12.5.

12.4   CONCLUSIONS

We used the dataset available on the UCI Repository for training deep learning models to perform classification for two categorical classes, sober and intoxicated persons, using accelerometer values extracted from a smartphone sensor. This data was consistent with other studies on similar backgrounds, provided the true intoxication levels were already known in advance using the TAC sensors. We also acknowledged extremely useful features to be inspected in further studies of the research work. In this research process, we examined the relative value of automatic smartphone sensors and manually provided information. We first used familiar definitions of heavy drinking in alcohol research to assign heavy or non-heavy drinking labels for each night in the

TABLE 12.1
Model Result for Different People

Classifiers	LSTM	Bidirectional LSTM	ConvLSTM
MC7070	88.44	86.73	90.14
CC6740	81.09	83.42	87.69
DC6359	83.54	84.59	87.92
JB316	81.92	82.79	86.37
MJ8002	85.76	84.48	89.21
PC6771	83.68	84.17	87.84
SA0297	82.97	85.96	86.26
HV6018	82.74	82.86	87.29

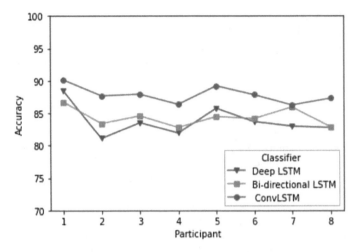

FIGURE 12.5 Comparison between the accuracy of various classifiers.

dataset for each person. We then established a deep learning model to classify this and compare the classification power of automatically captured sensor data versus manually contributed context information and images. The results obtained from the model are astonishing. We believe that our work has implications for alcohol research and potential applications related to self-tracking and health interventions.

12.5 FUTURE WORK AND IMPROVEMENTS

Even though we attained incredible accuracy for different people, we saw some challenges in our study. First, not regulating for phone situation enabled us to capture more general use cases. Suppose data from gyroscope is used and combined with the accelerometer data. In that case, the accuracy can be improved by considering the phone's movement and the direction in which it is oriented. Moreover, with more data from the sensor, more engagement with data must include the phone's alignment before arrangements recover.

Moreover, we took random subject's motions for whom it could be hard to learn common arrangement instructions. This might be improved by converging a type of motion, such as a walking event. We tried to look at mobile events after their processing but found a decline in accuracy. Via a phone's integral procedure for fading data of walking at sensor-time could be a promising direction. This proposes that more compound methods or features capable of showing the varied user actions in drinking heavily might be needed for further improvement.

REFERENCES

1. SAMHSA. *2018 National Survey on Drug Use and Health. Table 7.16A—Alcohol Use in Lifetime, Past Year, and Past Month among Persons Aged 12 to 20, by Gender: Numbers in Thousands, 2002–2018.*

2. SAMHSA. *2018 National Survey on Drug Use and Health. Table 7.16B—Alcohol Use in Lifetime, Past Year, and Past Month among Persons Aged 12 or Older, by Detailed Age Category: Percentages, 2017 and 2018.*

3. Hingson, R.W., Zha, W., Weitzman, E.R. "Magnitude of and trends in alcohol-related mortality and morbidity among US college students ages 18–24, 1998–2005," *Journal of Studies on Alcohol and Drugs*, (Suppl. 16), 12–20, 2009, PMID: 19538908.

4. Hingson, R., Heeren, T., Winter, M. et al. "Magnitude of alcohol-related mortality and morbidity among US college students ages 18–24: Changes from 1998 to 2001," *Annual Review of Public Health*, 26, 2005, 259–279. PMID: 15760289.

5. DeJong, W., Larimer, M.E., Wood, M.D., Hartman, R. "NIAAA's rapid response to college drinking problems initiative: reinforcing the use of evidence-based approaches in college alcohol prevention," *Journal of Studies on Alcohol and Drugs*, supplement, 16, 2009, 5–11.

6. Brown-Rice, Kathleen A., Furr, Susan, Jorgensen, Maribeth. "Analysing Greek members alcohol consumption by gender and the impact of alcohol education interventions," *Journal of Alcohol and Drug Education*, 59(1), 2015, 19–38.

7. Borsari, Brian, Carey, Kate B. "Effects of a brief motivational intervention with college student drinkers," *Journal of Consulting and Clinical Psychology*, 68(4), 2000, 728.

8. Thompson, E.B., Heley, F., Oster-Aaland, L., Stastny, S.N., Crawford, E.C. "The impact of a student-driven social marketing campaign on college student alcohol-related beliefs and behaviors," *Social Marketing Quarterly*, 19(1), 2013, 52–64.

9. Carey, Kate B., Hustad, John T.P. "Methods for determining blood alcohol concentration: Current and retrospective," in *Comprehensive handbook of alcohol related pathology*, 2005. Elsevier Inc, pp. 1429–1444.

10. Kelly, Sarah, Olanrewaju, Olawale, Cowan, Andy, Brayne, Carol, Lafortune, Louise. "Interventions to prevent and reduce excessive alcohol consumption in older people: a systematic review and meta-analysis," *Age and Ageing*, 47(2), 2018, 175–184.

11. Lee, John D., Fiorentino, Dary, Reyes, Michelle L., Brown, Timothy L., Ahmad, Omar, Fell, James, Ward, Nic, Dufour, Robert. *Assessing the feasibility of vehicle-based sensors to detect alcohol impairment*, year??. National Highway Traffic Safety Administration.

12. Nyman, E., Palmlöv, A. (1936). The Elimination of Ethyl Alcohol in Sweat 1. *Skandinavisches Archiv Für Physiologie*, 74(2), 2010, 155–159.

13. Swift, Robert M., Martin, Christopher S., Swette, Larry, LaConti, Anthony, Kackley, Nancy. "Studies on a wearable, electronic, transdermal alcohol sensor," *Alcoholism: Clinical and Experimental Research*, 16(4), 1992, 721–725.

14. Hardeman, Wendy, Houghton, Julie, Lane, Kathleen, Jones, Andy, Naughton, Felix. "A systematic review of just-in-time adaptive interventions (JITAIs) to promote physical activity," *International Journal of Behavioral Nutrition and Physical Activity*, 16(1), 2019, 31.

15. Nahum-Shani, Inbal, Smith, Shawna N., Spring, Bonnie J., Collins, Linda M., Witkiewitz, Katie, Tewari, Ambuj, Murphy, Susan A. "Just-in-time adaptive interventions (JITAIs) in mobile health: key components and design principles for ongoing health behavior support," *Annals of Behavioral Medicine*, 52(6), 2018, 446–462.

16. Killian, J.A., Passino, K.M., Nandi, A., Madden, D.R. Clapp, J. "Learning to Detect Heavy Drinking Episodes Using Smartphone Accelerometer Data," in *Proceedings of the 4th International Workshop on Knowledge Discovery in Healthcare Data co-located with the 28th International Joint Conference on Artificial Intelligence*, 2019. IJCAI, pp. 35–42.

17. Gers, Felix A., Eck, Douglas, Schmidhuber, Jürgen. "Applying LSTM to time series predictable through time-window approaches," in *Neural Nets WIRN Vietri-01*, 2002. Springer, pp. 193–200.

18. Kaushik, Shruti, Choudhury, Abhinav, Sheron, Pankaj Kumar, Dasgupta, Nataraj, Natarajan, Sayee, Pickett, Larry A., Dutt, Varun. "AI in healthcare: time-series forecasting using statistical, neural, and ensemble architectures," *Frontiers in Big Data*, 3, 2020, 4.

19. Karim, Fazle, Majumdar, Somshubra, Darabi, Houshang, Chen, Shun. "LSTM fully convolutional networks for time series classification," *IEEE Access*, 6, 2017, 1662–1669.

20. Tan, Hui Xing, Aung, Nway, Tian, Jing, Chin, Matthew, Heng, Chua, Yang, Youheng Ou. "Time series classification using a modified LSTM approach from accelerometer-based data: A comparative study for gait cycle detection," *Gait & Posture*, 74, 2019, 128–134.

21. Hochreiter, Sepp, Schmidhuber, Jürgen. "Long short-term memory," *Neural Computation*, 9(8), 1997, 1735–1780.

22. Javaid, Ali, Zafar, Afia, Ahemed, Zaheer. "A Review On Techniques For Water Quality Monitoring Using IoT Devices," *Big Data In Water Resources Engineering (BDWRE)*, 1(2), 2020, 49–51.

23. Guan, Yu, Plötz, Thomas. "Ensembles of deep lstm learners for activity recognition using wearables," *Proceedings of the ACM on Interactive, Mobile, Wearable and Ubiquitous Technologies*, 1(2), 2017, 1–28.

24. Zhu, Wentao, Lan, Cuiling, Xing, Junliang, Zeng, Wenjun, Li Shen, Yanghao, Xie, Xiaohui. "Co-occurrence feature learning for skeleton based action recognition using regularised deep LSTM networks," *arXiv preprint arXiv:1603.07772*, 2016.

25. Eyobu Odongo, Steven, Han, Dong Seog. "Feature representation and data augmentation for human activity classification based on wearable IMU sensor data using a deep LSTM neural network," *Sensors*, 18(9), 2018, 2892.

26. Malki, Zohair, Atlam, Elsayed, Dagnew, Guesh, Alzighaibi, Ahmad Reda, Ghada, Elmarhomy, Gad, Ibrahim. "Bidirectional Residual LSTM-based Human Activity Recognition," *Computer and Information Science*, 13(3), 2020, 1–40.

27. Chen, Zhu, Wu, Bangyu, Li, Bin, Ruan, Housong. "Expressway Exit Traffic Flow Prediction for ETC and MTC Charging System Based on Entry Traffic Flows and LSTM Model," *IEEE Access*, 9, 2021, 54613–54624.

28. Hernández, Fabio, Suárez, Luis F., Villamizar, Javier, Altuve, Miguel. "Human activity recognition on smartphones using a bidirectional lstm network," in *2019 XXII Symposium on Image, Signal Processing and Artificial Vision (STSIVA)*, 2019. IEEE, pp. 1–5.

29. Li, Wenhui, Nie, Weizhi, Su, Yuting. "Human action recognition based on selected spatio-temporal features via bidirectional LSTM," *IEEE Access*, 6, 2018, 44211–44220.

30. Li, Pei, Abdel-Aty, Mohamed, and Yuan, Jinghui. "Real-time crash risk prediction on arterials based on LSTM-CNN," *Accident Analysis & Prevention*, 135, 2020, 105371.

31. Qiao, Huihui, Wang, Taiyong, Wang, Peng, Qiao, Shibin, Zhang, Lan. "A time-distributed spatiotemporal feature learning method for machine health monitoring with multi-sensor time series," *Sensors*, 18(9), 2018, 2932.

32. Liu, Yipeng, Zheng, Haifeng, Feng, Xinxin, Chen, Zhonghui. "Short-term traffic flow prediction with Conv-LSTM," in *2017 9th International Conference on Wireless Communications and Signal Processing (WCSP)*, 2017. IEEE, pp. 1–6.

33. Xu, Cheng, Chai, Duo, He, Jie, Zhang, Xiaotong, Duan, Shihong. "InnoHAR: a deep neural network for complex human activity recognition," *IEEE Access*, 7, 2019, 9893–9902.

34. Hara, Kazuyuki, Saito, Daisuke, Shouno, Hayaru. "Analysis of function of rectified linear unit used in deep learning," in *2015 International Joint Conference on Neural Networks (IJCNN)*, 2015. *IEEE*, pp. 1–8.

Unit 4

*Security and Privacy in
IoT-Based Systems for
Healthcare Sector*

Unit 4

13 Cyber Security for Handling Threats in Healthcare Devices

Reshu Agarwal
Amity Institute of Information Technology
Amity University

Mukul Kumar
G.L. Bajaj Institute of Technology and Management

CONTENTS

DOI: 10.1201/9781003146087-17

Cybersecurity is the technique to protect networks, devices, and data from unauthorised access. It has been observed that some threats like data theft, phishing, and scams are greatly increasing day by day. As a developing innovation, the Internet of Things (IoT) has altered the worldwide organisation involving individuals, smart devices, intelligent objects, information, and data. In healthcare, IoT offers numerous advantages. When we integrate IoT with healthcare equipment, the prime concern is to provide risk-free treatment. Glucose meters, blood pressure cuffs, and other equipment are used to record patient vital signs and allow healthcare providers to collect information automatically.

But on the contrary, they neglect the factor of security, which emerges by connecting devices to the internet. A possibility of zero-day misuse in healthcare equipment can be misused for causing any injuries or even killing someone without even being traced. The improvement of IoT Healthcare systems is still at its outset, and many related issues should be settled. Device makers should be able to manage cyber vulnerabilities. In this chapter, we look to find the role of the IoT in healthcare, vulnerabilities, attack, and security issues and solutions.

13.1   INTRODUCTION

IoT acts as a network of physical devices that are both connected and intelligent. These devices comprise software, sensors, network connectivity that helps in collecting and exchanging data. IoT can be put into effect remotely across the existing network infrastructure, which paves the way for more direct integration of the device into a computer-based system, resulting in better efficiency and accuracy. In healthcare, the "things" of the Internet of Things is used to describe a wide variety of devices, such as heart-monitoring implants infusion pumps used in hospitals to deliver a pre-programmed level of fluids inpatient. There are very man other devices present, like pacemakers, insulin pumps, and cochlear implants. Few of these devices are used to transfer information with the help of a wireless connection like a pacemaker; on the other hand, other devices can send and receive data. IoT provides the healthcare sector with the opportunity to redefine and re-create the way things are done. And, in addition, there always exist different ways as to how these devices are secured and protected. For better safety and reliability of these healthcares, some security factors must be considered. Data and information hacking is very common these days. Hence, all must understand the challenges of cybersecurity. It is a technique to protect networks, devices, and data in cyberspace. It is related to the internet. Cybersecurity is the detection, analysis, and reduction in the possibility of being attacked or harmed in today's computer-based virtual environment. Due to globalisation, global networks and computer devices are exponentially increasing. There are three fundamental terms that are critical for cybersecurity: confidentiality, integrity, and availability.

Confidentiality: Data that is error-prone or confidential must remain so and is imparted just to constrained clients.
Integrity: Data must be consistent and not be changed from its unique state.
Availability: Information and frameworks must be accessible only to suitable clients.

Cyber attacks can be classified into several types, which depend on the nature of the hacker's information. This chapter includes the role of IoT in healthcare and explores associated attacks, vulnerabilities, security issues, and suggests solutions.

13.2   LITERATURE SURVEY

Many types of research have been done in the field of cybersecurity. These are based on every situation of management of cybersecurity. Cybercafes play a vital role in providing internet service as a shared access point. They act effectively in bridging the digital divide for the middle-class people in developing countries. Many researchers focus on the fact that cybercafes should not be distinguished based on caste, age, sectors, and other factors [1], [3], [7]. According to studies, it has been observed that internet cafes have played the lead role in changing lifestyle of youth. The use of internet cafes, along with the absence of social exercises, are contributory factord the in the decline in youth mental health.

Another measurement has been proposed concentrating on growing illicit apartments and social practices [4], [27], [29]. The outline of cyber crime and its effects helps in recognising the future pattern of cyber violations and the digital wrongdoings into various parts.

In cyber crime, preventive measures and existing laws were not powerful enough to check digital violations. More recently, other explorations have been carried on computer-related illicit acts and instruments and systems [5], [26]. A few analysts told about different violations, such as computer crimes and different cyber crime information system violations. They have likewise given a halfway perspective of the data frame, which can be actualised with the help of the UN. Later, the research was extended to discuss the types of cyber crimes and the way to handle such crimes using biometric techniques [6], [30]. Many cyber crimes use email spoofing, link manipulation, graphical substitution, DNS cache poisoning, and pharming. The one-time secret key has become an imperfective part of security on all shopping and other transactions to overcome this problem, as it assures information security and data assurance.

The one time secret key framework model can be used for verifying the account and opening documents [7]. A large portion of the research was working on this topic. This research are based on encoded OTP framework and its requirement in daily life. They were clarified as distinctive techniques and scientific equations for generating OTP [8]. Encrypted OTP in the mobile system and how we can use it to protect our data was explained. Created OTP was sent through an SMS mechanism to the customer's mobile a record check. It is imperative for mobile banking or money-involved online transactions. The distinctive threat may happen in generating and exchanging OTP, and, in addition, diverse strategies for securing OTP was suggested by many researchers. Later the generation of the OTP system was described. A genetic algorithm with an elliptic curve cryptography procedure was utilised to produce another secret key for each transaction [9]. The loss of old secret keys is not an issue. We can obtain a new secret key, which results in an increment of our framework or activity security. Diverse procedures to safeguard the OTP from attackers were developed, and synchronisation issues while obtaining the OTP were terminated. Next, OTP generation is created by utilising SHA (Secure Hash Algorithm) calculation which produces new OTP inevitably. It likewise gave a new way to deal with OTP confirmation which gave additional security to our OTP [10], [28].

Further IoT solutions have extra limitations that must be fulfilled for complete health care solutions. These incorporate specialised (low preparing capacity, power-constrained, irregular correspondences) and client requirements (how does a patient with physical as well as mental challenges design and update their gadgets). Considering these challenges, Poyner and Sherratt [11] developed a framework for the secure and safe requirements for smart healthcare. Saha et al. [12] suggested an e-medical care structure that manages electronic clinical records (EMRs), saving privacy issues. Moreover, they compared this research with other recent works in terms of response time and delay. Results recommend that the proposed system is productive in giving security along with standard network parameters. Zhou and Piramuthu [13] proposed a method to address identified vulnerabilities. Abuladel and Bamasag [14] attended to the difficulties regarding IoT applications, focusing on client's information and area protection. Likewise, they contemplated two case situations of IoT clients in well-being applications. Both situations feature information and area security issues of IoT clients. Latif and Zafar [15] surveyed issues concerned with security and privacy in IoT appliances in developed cities.

Further, the Internet of Medical Things (IoMT) has become an expert application structure in the medical sector. It is used to aggregate and analyse the physiological limits of patients, to break down the clinical sensor hubs, which are embedded in the patient's body. It would hence distinguish the patient's clinical information using brilliant compact gadgets. Since the patient information is so sensitive to reveal to others, the security confirmation and insurance of clinical data are beconing a troublesome issue for IoMT. Deebak, Al-Turjman, Aloqaily and Alfandi [16] proposed a model to solve the above problem using a biometric-based user validation approach to ensure safe communication in medical appliances. Chaudhari and Umamaheswari [17] surveyed different models of healthcare based on the IoT to collect information on privacy and security issues. A significant number of plain issues need an answer. Ranjith and Mahantesh [18] made a precise review of various techniques and approaches utilised by analysts to actualise smart and secure healthcare. Sun et al. [19] proposed a model for healthcare in which users can encrypt and decrypt details regarding their personal use.

Further, accomplishing a quick information transfer rate is becoming more of an issue, given the huge amount of information delivered by the IoT devices. Bosri, et al. [20] proposed a framework based on blockchain technology to provide security. Tang et al. [21] proposed a health information aggregation scheme that safely gathers health information from different sources and guarantees reasonable motivations for contributing patients. Ahanger and Aljumah [22] proposed a model for recognising security issues related to the IoT networks to comprehend the security necessities of IoT associations. Results recommend that security threats are one of the greatest issue for IoT. Therefore, it is essential to reduce them altogether for the accomplishment of this stage. Alabdulatif et al. [24] introduced a solution for the above problem based on edge computing for providing more security for smart healthcare systems. The real challenge lies in the fact that composite IoT systems maintains security levels with new laws and regulations. To solve this problem, Amato et al. [25] proposed a model that utilises both work process dialects and semantics to engage the endorsement of the security features offered by a composite IoT system. Moreover, they keep in mind that the above solution should follow national and international laws also.

13.3   IOT AND ITS APPLICATIONS

Today, IoT is an important technology, attracting the attention of researchers. IoT represents a scheme consisting of a wired or wireless network structure. IoT sensors can use different types of connections. In addition to supporting RFID, Wi-Fi, Bluetooth, ZigBee, remote connection, various technologies like GSM, GPS etc., are possible. IOT enabled objects can share information among all peoples. The numerous uses of IoT promise to make life simpler and increasingly secure. There are numerous applications, for example, brilliant city, lodging, transportation, vitality, keen condition and so forth.

13.3.1   SMART HEALTHCARE

Before the appearance of IoT, communication between specialists and patients was simply through visits, writing, and telecommunications. There were no ways to empower specialists to screen their patients consistently and make proposals as needs arose. The development of IoT in medicinal services has extensively changed the scenario. It has engaged specialists to convey standout care by remotely checking patients utilising IoT-empowered devices. Moreover, IoT has likewise expanded the pace of fulfilment and commitment of patients as collaborating with specialists has become progressively agreeable and efficient. IoT has unarguably changed the social insurance industry and is exceptionally valuable for specialists, patients, families, emergency clinics, and even insurance agencies. However, numerous individuals on the planet, who are genuinely sick, do not have simple access to powerful medicinal services, so this is a significant weakness. Be that as it may, small but ground-breaking remote arrangements associated with IoT have made it conceivable to monitor these patients. These arrangements can be utilised to safely gather persistent well-being information from different sensors, apply entangled information investigation calculations, and offer remote association with human services experts who can make proper suggestions.

13.3.2 SMART CITY

An intelligent city can be thought of as a city of things to come and scholarly life. Following the smart urban development innovation rate, it will be possible to use IoT technology further in the future. It connects all cities, such as transportation systems, medical systems, and climate control systems, and allows people access to airports, railways, and airport databases. The demand for smart city needs cautious planning at each stage, by way of the support of the government and citizens, to implement IoT technology in all aspects.

13.3.3 SMART ENERGY

Intelligent networks are linked with information and control as they are being developed for intelligent energy management. An intelligent network that integrates information and communication technology (ICT) into a power grid enables real-time bidirectional communication between suppliers and consumers, allows for more active interactions in power flows, and provides efficient and sustained possible power. An important element of ICT is detecting and monitoring technology for energy flow and digital communication infrastructure for sending data over the network. Many applications can be operated through the internet for smart grid such as industry, solar, nuclear power, vehicle, hospital, urban energy control etc.

13.3.4 SMART GRID

The current network is extremely dependable and can withstand the normal fluctuation of power. It will make a stride towards a low-carbon vitality framework that empowers the incorporation of sustainable power sources. The special attention necessary for hospital patients whose physiological conditions need to be continuously monitored can be achieved using IoT monitoring techniques. Brilliant well-being sensors are utilised to gather total physiological data and dissect and store that data utilising portals and mists. Next, the broken down information is remotely transmitted to a medical attendant; further investigation and examination are then performed. Rather than giving a mechanised constant progression of data, it is an option in contrast to the procedure of consistently counselling a social insurance expert to confirm the patient's indispensable signs.

13.3.5 SMART TRANSPORTATION

Road condition monitoring and alerting applications are one of the most important applications of IoT conversion. Intelligent transport corresponds to three main concepts – transport analysis, transport control, and vehicle connection. Routing and vehicle speed control are closely related to vehicle connection (V2X communication) in adding to traffic management and are regulated worldwide as transport control provided through multiple technologies. IoT can likewise be utilised for transportation – electric vehicles, a significant method to decrease fuel costs and worldwide temperature change, are creating extraordinary interest from drivers. In numerous nations, the legislature has bolstered for lithium-particle (Li-on) batteries for electric vehicles. The proposed scheme was developed to recognise the function of Li-ion batteries so that drivers can derive the driving situation from the actual driving conditions, and the driver can know the state of the road. This solution has been integrated with many important functions such as dynamic Li-on battery testing, online debugging, and remote monitoring with error correction, significantly reducing maintenance costs.

13.3.6 SMART FACTORY AND SMART MANUFACTURING

The astute processing plant generally changes how an item is fabricated and conveyed. Simultaneously, it has improved profitability, low emanations, and helps safeguard the planet. Creation will be more brilliant because of advances in how machines and different articles collaborate and adjust individuals' perspectives to the specialised framework. Expository prospects are provided by the totality and variety of information produced by arranged economies to upgrade mechanical procedures. The industrial revolution and manufacturing revolution have gotten one of the most trendsetting innovations.

13.4 IOT CHALLENGES

The fact of the IoT and its utilisation is very interesting as it provides intelligent technology for everything. The only challenge in applying concept of IoT in every field is in terms of underlying cost. You should be able to use technology with many objects at a low cost. IoT also faces many challenges.

13.4.1 SCALABILITY

The IoT is a big concept like a conventional internet computer. Therefore, basic functions such as communication and service discovery should work equally well in small and large environments. However, IoT requires new functions and methods to achieve efficient scalability.

13.4.2 AMOUNT OF DATA

In some IoT application scenarios, communication is infrequent; collecting large or shape-based sensor networks collects large amounts of data on nodes or centralised network servers. There is a large amount of data that requires many operation mechanisms and new technologies of memory, processing, and management.

13.4.3 DATA INTERPRETATION

To assist users of intelligent objects, it is necessary to interpret the local context as determined by the sensor as accurately as possible. Furthermore, for the service provider to benefit from the different data generated, generalised conclusions must be drawn from the interpreted sensor data.

13.4.4 AUTOMATIC DISCOVERY

In a dynamic environment, you need to automatically identify object-oriented services. To do that, you need appropriate semantic means to describe that function.

13.4.5 SOFTWARE COMPLEXITY

To manage intelligent objects and provide services that support intelligent objects, you need a larger network software infrastructure and a back-end server. This is because the smart object software system has to operate with minimum resources, as in conventional integrated systems.

13.4.6 SECURITY AND CONFIDENTIALITY

In addition to the internet security and protection aspects, such as communication confidentiality, communication partner reliability, and message integrity, other internet requirements are also important objects. For example, it is necessary to access specific services or avoid communication with others in IoT and even commercial transactions, including intelligent objects that need to be protect from competitors.

13.4.7 TOLERANCE

Internet objects are much more dynamic, mobile, and evolve unexpectedly faster than computers connected to the internet. Therefore, to build IoT robustly and reliably, we need multilevel redundancy and the ability to adapt automatically to changing conditions.

13.4.8 POWER SUPPLY

We anticipate a future low-power processor and an incorporated framework correspondence unit that can fundamentally decrease vitality utilisation. Vitality sparing is not just a component of equipment and framework engineering; it is likewise a programming component. For example, in the convention stack execution, each transmitted byte needs to legitimise its reality.

13.5 MEDJACKING: HOW HACKERS USE MEDICAL DEVICES TO LAUNCH CYBERATTACKS

13.5.1 MEDJACKING

According to a report by cybersecurity firm TrapX, hackers infect medical devices with malware and use them to launch cyber attacks on healthcare IT systems. According to case studies, hackers targeted at least three hospitals and infected the devices and equipment, resulting in a backdoor vulnerability called "medjack", i.e. medical device hijack.

   The first case involved an unnamed hospital where hackers planted malware in surgical blood gas analysers and used the equipment as a backdoor to get passwords throughout the hospital's IT system. In addition, they leaked some sensitive information out of the system and into the internet. Once the work is done, the vulnerability allows hackers to change unencrypted data stored inside the devices. In another case, the hospital's picture archive and communications systems, i.e. PACS, where all the images the CT scanners, MRI scanners, and X-Ray machines are stored, were used by hackers to get access into other parts of the hospital's database. In the third case, the hackers created the backdoor using the X-ray system.

The case study of TrapX mentioned that there are commonly used medical devices that are running out-of-date, closed, often modified, or less secure operating systems such as Windows 2000, XP, or Linux. As a result, the IT team in healthcare cannot access the outdated software installed in the systems. As a result, they become easy hacking targets and ideal points from which hackers can launch attacks to acquire sensitive information about patients and hospitals.

13.5.2 TYPES OF ATTACKS

- **Brute Force Attack**
- To get users' passwords and PINs (personal identification numbers), various automated software can harm the system by generating various guesses of desired data. These data can be obtained using trial and error methods. This type of attack will use distinctively designed software to break the password by entering thousands of different words, strings, and numeric values.
- **Social Engineering/Cyber Fraud**
- The attackers are mainly acting against the system; they are attacking persons, groups of people, and companies' wire-transfer protocols and working methodology. This attack not only targets data; it is mostly aimed at a monetary target, and once it is executed, it is impossible to retrieve that monetary value.
- **Distributed Denial-of-Service Attack (DDoS)**
- The main effect of these attacks is heavy congestion on a specific server with multiple connections. It finally closes the attacked website or network system. Here attackers target the system and make it very congested to cause the network shut off, and preventing people from being able to work.
- **Phishing Attacks**
- Phishing is the most common attack and can be very difficult to resist. Phishing attacks are of many types, and depending on the company structure, different types are applied. Attackers send thousands of emails having URL links or an attachment with the aim that someone will open them. Then, with a single click on those links, attackers can access all the information present on the system, which may lead to attacks on software, loss of passwords, disabling firewalls, or intruding on security tools.
- **Ransomware, Malware and Spyware**
- All the attackers under this category have their own particular target. These may be attacks on computer systems, software, and malware-secured software – these attacks can affect and access the above systems very easily. This kind of threat generally impacts faulty software and can access such software in

an unauthorised way. They involve mostly viruses and spy software. Nowadays attackers can hack your system and lock it. They generally blackmail by restricting uses from access to important information, demanding a ransom to access the system again. The data or the information stored in the system can be damaged or removed if these viruses enter the system.

13.6 SECURING IOT IN HEALTHCARE

It has been accepted by all healthcare communities that IoT will be a part of their future. They know that digitising and streamlining health data sharing will help them gain more efficiency and be cost-efficient. But there should be some security steps that manufacturers and providers of IoT devices can take, including encryption and a secure boot. A secure boot ensures that once the device is turned on, there has not been any modification in the device's configurations. It is a challenge for those in charge of systems, as they still need to figure out how to manage the risks of IoT and use the benefits. The experts can take many steps to reduce IoT risks and capture the benefits, which include the following.

- **Inventory devices:** All assets should need to be taken into consideration as organisations cannot secure what they cannot see. For instance, an admitted patient can bring a Google Home or Alexa for entertainment use. Some tools in the market can detect IoT devices on the network without interrupting their functionalities. These tools can also identify which OS is running on the device.
- **Follow best practices:** experts should follow best security practices for healthcare IoT devices, such as the hard-coded passwords, encryption, and firewalls should be eliminated. A risk assessment should be done before any IoT devices are deployed in the hospital, thereby reducing vulnerabilities. All the devices present should be updated regularly.
- **Effective authentication:** Public key infrastructure and digital certificates can ensure authentic connections are made with the network and other devices. Also, it would ensure no manipulations are done to the data packages while in transit.
- **Segment networks:** The connectivity of some devices should be limited. For instance, if the device is meant for patient care, its capability to connect to the internet should be turned off. Healthcare organisations can work with vendors to know which connections are required and allow those connections, creating an allow list. There can also be a deny list that mentions all the harmful sites from which the connection should not be made. The public network should be segmented from the rest of the network and restrict access to assets and events on a virtual LAN.
- **Use the right tools:** Healthcare organisations should use tools that ensure the IoT devices' security. Some platforms can manage massive amounts of data and devices and can control authentication. Some devices can identify what a device is used for, what data is collected from it and where the connectivity lies.

13.7 HOW TO MANAGE RISKS ASSOCIATED WITH CYBERSECURITY

The risks related to any cyber attack rely upon three factors: threats, vulnerabilities, and impacts. Any malicious attempt to access a computer network without the owner's permission is termed a cyber threat. Cyber attack can be done within the organisation by trusted clients or by unknown people over the internet from remote areas. There are numerous wellsprings of dangers like threatening governments, terrorist groups, displeased representatives, and malicious intruders. Vulnerabilities simply allude to shortcomings in a framework. Vulnerabilities make dangers conceivable and possibly much riskier. A single vulnerability can put an entire framework at risk. For instance, delicate information can be effortlessly assaulted by a single SQL injection vulnerability. An attacker could chain a few adventures together, abusing more than one weakness to misuse a framework.

The effect of a cyber attack on any association leads to financial and reputational misfortune. An effective attack can trade off the secrecy, respectability, and accessibility of the framework and the data it handles. Now and again, the protected innovation of an organisation, like copyright, patents competitive advantage can be stolen, leading to greater misfortune. The data is very important and it should be protected; anyway, the loss of such data might harm relationships as contenders may use it. Information that is worth cash and is confidential needs to be safeguarded; however, loss of information will cause an immense warning to the organisation as it will profit competitors. Once any organisation faces any cyber attack, their clients do not feel safe with their information in that organisation. It will therefore lead the client to move to another organisation for services. By removing the threat sources, the risks of cyber attacks are managed. This can be done by reducing incentives for cyber criminals or by closing down botnets.

13.8 NECESSITY OF CYBERSECURITY

One of the most important factors for an individual, corporate sector as well as state is information. Cybersecurity is important because:

- It provides security to an individual's account from hijacking while using social networking sites.
- It prevents unauthorised access, disclosure, and modification of systems resources.
- It makes online transactions in banking, shopping, railway reservations etc., more secure.
- It imparts knowledge of the threat and of the vectors that attackers use to outwit cyber defences.

13.9 ENCRYPTION ALGORITHMS FOR ENHANCING CYBERSECURITY

- **Triple DES:** Triple DES was designed to take the native data encryption (DES) algorithm, which attackers easily defeated. TED is the most prominent algorithm used in industry. It makes use of three keys, each of 56 bits. According to experts, the key length adds up to 168 bits, but 112 bits in key strength is more likely.

- **RSA:** It is used to encrypt data sent over the internet. It is a public-key encryption algorithm, and GPG programs use RSA as one of their algorithms. Unlike Triple DES, RSA uses a pair of keys, so it is considered an asymmetric algorithm. The public key is used for encrypting, and the private key is used for decrypting messages. The outcome of RSA encryption includes a large number of mumbo jumbo, which takes attackers considerably more time and processing power to break.
- **Blowfish:** It was also designed to replace DES. It is a symmetric cypher that breaks messages into blocks of 64 bits and then encrypts them. This algorithm is popular for its speed and efficiency. It is said that it has never been defeated. Its free availability in the public domain makes it a good choice for vendors. Software categories like e-commerce platforms for securing payments and password managements tools make use of Blowfish. Blowfish is the most flexible encryption method available nowadays.
- **Twofish:** Blowfish and its successor Twofish is the brainchild of computer security expert Bruce Schneier. It is one of the fastest algorithms and is perfect for use in hardware and software environments. Twofish is also freely available, so it is widely found in encryption programs like PhotoEncrypt, CPG and popular open-source software TrueCrypt.
- **AES:** The AES stands for advanced encryption algorithm. The US government and numerous organisations trust it. It is most efficient in 12-bit form but uses 192 and 256 bits for heavy-duty encryption. It is unaffected by all the attacks, but brute force is an exception. It uses all combinations of 128, 192, and 256-bit cyphers to decipher messages. According to security experts, AES will be considered for encrypting data in the private sector.

13.10   ADVANCES IN CYBERSECURITY TECHNOLOGY

- **Artificial Intelligence and Deep Learning:** Two-factor authentication confirms the user's identity based on two to three parameters. Additional to this, for more layers of authentication and identity management, artificial intelligence is used. Deep learning is used for analysing data such as logs, transactions. Real-time communications are also analysed with deep learning techniques to detect threats and unwanted activities.
- **Behavioural Analytics:** It helps to discover designs on a framework and organisation exercises to recognise potential and constant threats. For example, a sudden increase from a user device can be a symptom of a possible cybersecurity issue. Although this technology is mostly used for networks, its application in systems and user devices has increased.
- **Blockchain Cybersecurity:** This is one of the most recent network protection innovations: acknowledgement and energy – the blockchain innovation capacities based on recognisable proof between the two exchange parties. Likewise,

blockchain cybersecurity works based on peer-to-peer network fundamentals. As a result, blockchain establishes near-impenetrable networks for hackers. Also, blockchain with AI results in a robust verification system to keep potential cyber threats at bay.

- **Zero-Trust Model:** This cybersecurity model is faced with the assumption that a network is already compromised. Due to this belief, one cannot trust the network; one would surely boost external and internal security. The essence of this strategy is that both the outside and the inside of the organisation is vulnerable to a trade-off and need the same level of insurance. It envelops recognising business-basic information, planning the stream of the business information, physical and intelligent division, and strategy and control implementation through robotisation and persistent observing.
- **Embedded Hardware Authentication:** Embedded authenticators are arising technologies to authenticate a user's identity by validating passwords and PINS. Intel has introduced sixth-generation vPro Chips in this domain. These chips are embedded in the hardware itself and provide powerful user identification.

13.11   CYBERETHICS

Cyberethics refers to a code of behaviour or set of morals applied to the online environment – these ethics result in making cyberspace a safer place. When we follow these ethics, it ensures that we are utilising the web appropriately and more securely. Standard Cyberethics are as follows:

- Do not be a bully on the internet.
- Never access other's account utilising their credentials.
- Never endeavour to send any malware or harmful messages to other systems as it ends, resulting in their system corruption.
- Always adhere to copyrighted information.
- Never share your personal information with unknown people over the internet, as this gives the attacker a good chance to misuse your information and lead to trouble.
- Respect all other internet users. Do not threaten, harass, stalk or abuse anyone.
- Do not store, send, or disseminate any content that can be offensive to a reasonable person.
- Be a law-abiding and responsible internet user.

13.12   RECENT SURVEY ISSUES IN CYBERSECURITY

- **Mobile Computing**: Mobile computing is a growing field in the age of cybersecurity. The exponential growth in security risks is due to an exponential growth of mobile devices. Each new smartphone, tablet, or other cell phone creates another powerless access point to systems and opens another window for a digital assault.

- **Social Media Networking:** Cyber threats are caused because of the exceptional expansion of online networking. The application of online networking within organisations is a rapidly increasing threat. In 2020, it can be expected that there would be a great expansion in the field of online networking profiles for social designing strategies. To minimise the security threat within organisations, there should be propelled advancements, such as information leakage prevention, improved system checking, and log record examination with improved approaches and methods.
- **Cloud Computing:** Cloud computing offers end clients the advantage of virtually unlimited computing resources, the accommodation of expert framework activity and support, and the economy of on-request billing. Security-based risks are mostly involved with cloud computing. Clouds generally consist of multiple entities, which means that no configuration can be more secure than its weakest link. There can be simultaneous attacks on multiple sites due to the link between separate entities. Clouds become a target for cyber criminals when cloud providers do not employ adequate cybersecurity measures.

13.13   SCOPE OF AI IN CYBERSECURITY

AI has many potentials, and companies need to access this potential and use it in cybersecurity infrastructure. AI enhances cybersecurity with an absorbed focus on outreach. Some researchers have revealed that 64% of all alerts are overlooked, and only 23% of companies react to them during a crisis. The nature of cybersecurity needs to be changed so that a comprehensive approach can be built to security management. It means that we need to lay more emphasis on AI in cybersecurity. With the introduction of a new tool and sophisticated algorithms, it will be interesting to see who has a broader reach. AI can scan a whole systems' file and find out the threats in advance; this capability of AI takes the entire ecosystem to another much more enhanced level . Because AI works based on feedback, it provides more scope to teams at large. Many tools are available to cyber teams, who can then feed that data back into AI algorithms. This makes the system more robust and paves the path for machine-learning integration. Nowadays nearly 20% of C-Suite executives are making use of machine learning to amplify their AI offerings, so there is a need to strengthen the scope of AI and its reach. AI needs to evolve in such a way that it has a wider view and a more rational process when it comes to threat detection.

13.14   CONCLUSION AND FUTURE SCOPE

Cybersecurity means to secure data and its frameworks by utilising the right safety methods. For security to personal information and PC systems, using a firewall and antivirus is common, but they do not ensure complete security. This chapter has reviewed cybersecurity in various fields. Each basic framework likewise needs digital security rather than physical security or any other kind of security. Each segment utilises diverse strategies to give digital security to an association, as we discussed above. IoMT is growing tremendously and promises to advance patient engagement and provide better healthcare facilities. Although IoMT has numerous advantages, it poses certain security risks. Healthcare IT managers and chief information security officers should be aware of the risks posed and should take the required steps and monitor deployed IoT technology to eliminate cyber risks. In future, there is scope for more scientific methodologies that can be integrated into cybersecurity to incorporate various security challenges. Cyber security is a continuous changing process that requires regular work and training to maintain a secure infrastructure. It is impossible to consider a system 100% secure and risk-free. To sustain a secure environment, continuous monitoring and advancement of security methods in healthcare are needed.

REFERENCES

1. Khan, M.H. "OTP Generation using SHA," *International Journal on Recent and Innovation Trends in Computing and Communication*, 3(4), 2015, 2244–2245.
2. Ahlawat, P., Nandlal, R. "A Survey: Novel Approach Secure Authentication Technique by One Time Password using Mobile SMS," *International Journal of Enhanced Research in Science Technology & Engineering*, 4(6), 2015, 145–148.
3. Haseloff, A.M. "Cybercafes and their Potential as Community Development Tools in India," *Journal of Community Informatics*, 1(3), 2005, 14–21.
4. Saini, H., Rao, Y.S., Panda, T.C. "Cyber Crimes and their Impacts: A Review," *International Journal of Engineering Research and Applications*, 2(2), 2012, 202–209.
5. Kandpal, V., Singh, R.K. "Latest Face of Cybercrime and Its Prevention In India," *International Journal of Basic and Applied Sciences*, 2(4), 2013, 150–156.
6. Puthenkovilakam, J. "Malicious attack detection and prevention in ad hoc network based on real time operating system environment," *International Journal of Research in Engineering and Technology*, 2(6), 2013, 1043–1046.
7. Ahlawat, P., Nandlal, R. "A Survey: Novel Approach Secure Authentication Technique by One Time Password using Mobile SMS," *International Journal of Enhanced Research in Science Technology & Engineering*, 4(6), 2015, 145–148.
8. Shrivastava, S. "Rushing Attack and its Prevention Techniques," *International journal of application and innovation in engineering and management*, 2(4), 2013, 453–456.
9. Huang, Y., Huang, Z., Zhao, H., Lai, X. "A new One-time Password Method," *IERI Procedia*, 4, 2014, 32–37, https://doi.org/10.1016/j.ieri.2013.11.006.
10. Gross, M.L., Canetti, D., Vashdi, D.R. "Cyberterrorism: its effects on psychological well-being, public confidence and political attitudes," *Journal of Cybersecurity*, 3(1), 2017, 49–58.
11. Poyner, K. and Sherratt, R.S. "Privacy and security of consumer IoT devices for the pervasive monitoring of vulnerable people," *Living in the Internet of Things: Cybersecurity of the IoT*, 2018, 1–5, doi: 10..1049/cp.2018.0043.
12. Saha, R., Kumar, G., Rai, M.K., Thomas, R., Lim, S. "Privacy Ensured e-Healthcare for Fog-Enhanced IoT Based Applications," *IEEE Access*, 7(1), 2019, 44536–44543, doi: 10.1109/ACCESS.2019.2908664.
13. Zhou, W., Piramuthu, S. "Security/privacy of wearable fitness tracking IoT devices," *9th Iberian Conference on Information Systems and Technologies (CISTI), Barcelona, Spain*, 2014, 1–5, doi: 10.1109/CISTI.2014.6877073.
14. Abuladel, A, Bamasag, O. "Data and Location Privacy Issues in IoT Applications," *3rd International Conference on Computer Applications & Information Security (ICCAIS)*, 2020, 1–6, doi: 10.1109/ICCAIS48893.2020.9096837.

15. Latif, S., Zafar, N.A. "A survey of security and privacy issues in IoT for smart cities," *Fifth International Conference on Aerospace Science & Engineering (ICASE)*, 2017, 1–5, doi: 10.1109/ICASE.2017.8374288.

16. Deebak, B.D., Al-Turjman, F., Aloqaily, M, Alfandi, O. "An Authentic-Based Privacy Preservation Protocol for Smart e-Healthcare Systems in IoT, *IEEE Access*," 7, 2019, 135632–135649, doi: 10.1109/ACCESS.2019.2941575.

17. Chaudhari, D.A., Umamaheswari, E. "Survey on Data Management for Healthcare Using Internet of Things," *Fourth International Conference on Computing Communication Control and Automation (ICCUBEA)*, 2018, 1–7, doi: 10.1109/ICCUBEA.2018.8697556.

18. Ranjith, J., Mahantesh, K. (2019). "Privacy and Security issues in Smart Health Care," *4th International Conference on Electrical, Electronics, Communication, Computer Technologies and Optimization Techniques (ICEECCOT)*, 2019, 378–383, doi: 10.1109/ICEECCOT46775.2019.9114681.

19. Sun, J., Xiong, H., Liu, X., Zhang, Y., Nie, X., Deng, R.H. "Lightweight and Privacy-Aware Fine-Grained Access Control for IoT-Oriented Smart Health," *IEEE Internet of Things Journal*, 7(7), 2020, 6566–6575, doi: 10.1109/JIOT.2020.2974257.

20. Bosri, R., Uzzal, A.R., Al Omar, A., Bhuiyan, M.Z.A., Rahman, M.S. "HIDEchain: A User-Centric Secure Edge Computing Architecture for Healthcare IoT Devices," *IEEE Conference on Computer Communications Workshops (INFOCOM WKSHPS)*, 2020, 376–381, doi: 10.1109/INFOCOMWKSHPS50562.2020.9162729.

21. Tang, W., Ren, J., Deng, K., Zhang, Y. "Secure Data Aggregation of Lightweight E-Healthcare IoT Devices With Fair Incentives," *IEEE Internet of Things Journal*, 6(5), 2019, 8714–8726, doi: 10.1109/JIOT.2019.2923261.

22. Ahanger, T.A., Aljumah, A. "Internet of Things: A Comprehensive Study of Security Issues and Defense Mechanisms," *IEEE Access*, 7, 2019, 11020–11028, doi: 10.1109/ACCESS.2018.2876939.

23. de Fuentes, J. Maria, Gonzalez-Manzano, L., Solanas, A., Veseli, F. "Attribute-Based Credentials for Privacy-Aware Smart Health Services in IoT-Based Smart Cities," *Computer*, 51(7), 2018, 44–53, doi: 10.1109/MC.2018.3011042.

24. Alabdulatif, A., Khalil, I., Yi, X., Guizani, M. "Secure Edge of Things for Smart Healthcare Surveillance Framework," *IEEE Access*, 7(1), 2019, 31010–31021, doi: 10.1109/ACCESS.2019.2899323.

25. Amato, F., Casola, V., Cozzolino, G., De Benedictis, A., Moscato, F. "Exploiting Workflow Languages and Semantics for Validation of Security Policies in IoT Composite Services," *IEEE Internet of Things Journal*, 7(5), 2020, 4655–4665, doi: 10.1109/JIOT.2019.2960316.

26. Mehta, S., Singh, S.D., Kumari, S., Karatangi, S.V., Agarwal, R., Rai, A. "Design and Implementation of Biometrically Activated Self-Defence Device for Women's Safety," in Mathur G., Sharma H., Bundele M., Dey N., Paprzycki M., *International Conference on Artificial Intelligence: Advances and Applications 2019. Algorithms for Intelligent Systems*, 2020. Springer. doi: https://doi.org/10.1007/978-981-15-1059-5_14.

27. Simplicio, M.A., Iwaya, LH., Barros, B.M., Carvalho, T.C.M.B., Näslund, M. "SecourHealth: A Delay-Tolerant Security Framework for Mobile Health Data Collection," *IEEE Journal of Biomedical and Health Informatics*, 19(2), 2015, 761–772, doi: 10.1109/JBHI.2014.2320444.

28. Tawalbeh, L.A., Tawalbeh, H., Song, H., Jararweh, Y. "Intrusion and attacks over mobile networks and cloud health systems," *IEEE Conference on Computer Communications Workshops (INFOCOM WKSHPS)*, 2017, 13–17, doi: 10.1109/INFCOMW.2017.8116345.

29. Shih, C., Chou, K., Keh, H., Cheng, Y., Yu, P., Huang, N. "Building Long-Distance Health Care Network Using Minimized Portable Sensors and Active Alert System," *16th International Conference on Network-Based Information Systems*, 2013, 401–404, doi: 10.1109/NBiS.2013.64.

30. Elkhodr, M., Shahrestani, S., Cheung, H. "Enhancing the security of mobile health monitoring systems through trust negotiations," *IEEE 36th Conference on Local Computer Networks*, 2011, 754–757, doi: 10.1109/LCN.2011.6115545.

29. Sun, [illegible] Building [illegible] Health Care [illegible] [illegible] Issues and [illegible] [illegible] *Informatics* [illegible]

30. [illegible] [illegible]

14 Security Challenges and Solutions for Healthcare in the Internet of Things

Bipin Kumar Rai
IT Department
ABES Institute of Technology

CONTENTS

The internet-based electronic health record (EHR) system allows patients to access remotely the required medical history whenever needed. Accessing patient records and the transactions associated with the diagnosis is beneficial for patients, the healthcare department, and executives. But this practice may lead to significant privacy concerns for the patient. No patient would like to reveal health-related data that may harm him/her or cause trouble in his/her personal and professional life. For EHR adaptation, the major elements are laws and regulations, monetary inducement and hurdles, technology state, and corporation effect. Emerging technologies like blockchain, cloud computing, the Internet of Things (IoT) have a vital role in healthcare information systems. This chapter discussed several privacy and security challenges and solutions for healthcare.

DOI: 10.1201/9781003146087-18

14.1 INTRODUCTION

EHR systems are greatly sought after for the structured unification of all pertinent medical data of an individual and to exhibit lifelong medical records. Various confidentiality threats of healthcare data are critical, either from within the institution or outside by some intruder. Each healthcare unit has an information system for maintaining patient data. Therefore, standards for data exchange are required, and EHRs and data needs to be standardised, including semantic interoperability (standards for the exchange of patient's data among EHR systems) [4]. Several solutions are available to create EHR standards, such as openEHR, Consolidated Health Informatics Initiative (CHI), Certification Commission for Healthcare Information Technology (CCHIT), Healthcare Information and Management Systems Society (HIMSS), American National Standards Institute (ANSI), and HL7 [11].

Google Health and Microsoft's HealthVault provide facility users to store and manage all health records in one central place. Anyone can import her/his health information from doctors, hospitals etc. Most of these services do not provide full control to the patients. Smart card healthcare systems developed in Europe are not strong at preserving privacy, as anyone can access a patient's information from a health card without her/his consent. Indivo is the first patient-controlled web-based healthcare system that provides options to own a secure complete medical record, integrating EHRs of different health centres.

An efficient protocol and architecture for EHRs are required, which is not standardised yet. EHR has succeeding advantages related to the cost-saving of adverse drug events, the collection of patient's healthcare data for research, and efficiency in medical treatment. Access control mechanisms and applications related to e-prescription systems and other consumer-related healthcare services require a secure mechanism [3][7][8][10].

As we know, with the huge size of patients' data, its management becomes difficult; hence big data technology and cloud computing are required [18]. In future, blockchain technology seems to be more appealing in the field of healthcare [17]. IoT technologies enable doctors/hospital authorities to be more watchful and retain close connection with the patients. IoT can be used for data collected from IoT devices, which can help physicians to identify the best treatment process for patients and reach expected outcomes [21].

14.2 ANONYMISATION

Disassociation techniques include anonymisation, which is used nowadays for security purposes. Anonymisation can be done using depersonalisation, which is nothing but the removal of identifying information from health records, such that it cannot be revert back in any situation.

Anonymisation is an important non-reversible approach in healthcare information security; hence pseudonymisation of medical data for privacy issues in healthcare is a central issue, but an efficient and acceptable approach is not available yet.

14.3 PSEUDONYMISATION

Pseudonymisation is most suitable for a healthcare information system which is similar to anonymisation. The only difference is that identifying information is separated from the health records, referenced by pseudonym (a unique random number) but not permanently deleted. Therefore, pseudonymisation is the patient-controlled reversible process under specified circumstances. Several mechanisms are available for ensuring security and privacy issues related to healthcare by pseudonymisation techniques [5][6][12–14].

Pseudonymisation techniques have the potential to handle the issue of identity management. It is also applied in several applications like healthcare information systems. Several mechanisms based on pseudonymisation are available to assure privacy and security issues related to EHR.

Pseudonymisation-based solutions for e-prescription systems are very appealing. Confidentiality and integrity of data are needed in a safe system, which the pseudonymisation technique can ensure.

14.4 ACCESS CONTROL

The access control objectives are protecting any information system from unauthorised access and at the same time making it available to authorised users [9]. EHR information systems need to develop a strong mechanism for protecting the unauthorised access of the data. The nature and constraints of the particular information system affect the access control methodology and architecture [15][16]. Whenever we think about the development of an access mechanism for EHR, the primary requirement is that it should be capable of satisfying the need of all entities like health centres, patients, doctors etc. For healthcare information systems, the following privacy and security requirements are crucial:

- Every healthcare entity should have the right to decide security policy and enforce it within its domain.
- The facility to healthcare providers to arbitrarily define the security of a particular document [9].
- Patients have control over their health records.
- The facility to the patient to grant access to certain medical practitioners.
- The feature for patients to delegate control of their health records to someone for emergencies.
- It should be simple to handle access control policies.

In the literature, three standard access control mechanisms have been recognised. Each standard was designed to solve limitations found in the previous one [1]:

(1) DAC (discretionary access control)
(2) MAC (mandatory access control)
(3) RBAC (role-based access control)

14.4.1 Discretionary Access Control

In DAC, each user accesses his/her data by his authorised identity. Its limitation are that:

(1) It is difficult to manage
(2) It might create new security issues.

14.4.2 Mandatory Access Control

- In the MAC mechanism, CA (Central Authority) decisions are made not by the owner of an object. The owner of data cannot change access rights.
- Medical personnel may assign access rights to a healthcare entity so some form of MAC policy should be involved.

Its limitations are:

(1) It is very difficult because of the huge number of users' medical records.
(2) It has limited scope because of unsuitability to patient control of their medical data.

14.4.3 Role-Based Access Control

Most of the existing access control mechanisms for the healthcare sector are either RBAC-based mechanisms or, in some sense, evolved from this mechanism. In RBAC, access to information is provided dependent on roles.
    Its limitation are:

(1) There is a central access control module, which the administrator could misuse.
(2) Some evaluations of access requests are complex as they need to consider contextual parameters.
(3) It is insufficient for the requirements of healthcare systems.

Access control mechanisms like DAC, MAC, and RBAC are insufficient for EHRs, but a combination of these can be used up to some extent.

14.4.4 Access Control Mechanism Suitable for Healthcare System

- **P-RBAC (Privacy-aware role-based access control)** is an extension of RBAC similar to XACML, which supports fine-grained policies. [10] shows a high-level specification of P-RBAC permissions support, an authoring tool based on the SPARCLE system.
- **Personalised access control** uses a combination of RBAC and DAC. In this approach the owner (the patient) will decide who can access her/his health data.

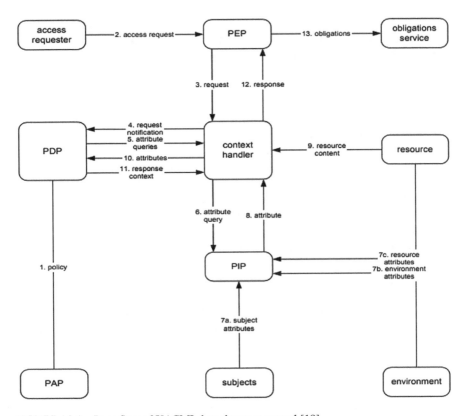

FIGURE 14.1 Data flow of XACML-based access control [19].

- **Context-related access control** for healthcare is RBAC with contextual parameters. It is not efficient to handle dynamic permission assignments.
- **Audit-based access control** is useful for an urgent situation. It allows the medical officer to handle exceptional situations and justify later.
- **Behaviour-based access control** is useful for handling the model compatible with several healthcare systems [1].
- **The rule-based access control approach** is for a resource-limited pervasive healthcare system [1].
- **XACML-based access control.** Figure 14.1 shows the sequence of steps.

14.5 E-HEALTH TRANSFORMATION MODEL IN SERBIA: DESIGN, ARCHITECTURE AND DEVELOPING

In Serbia, the architecture of the healthcare system is a hybrid smart card-based solution [2]. The database and two models, one online and the second offline, are briefly outlined here. In this system, RFID and IC-based smart cards have been used for national-level projects.

It includes an RFID antenna and microchip. Microchips can receive sufficient amounts of information. Chip cards are a kind of small computing machine that can perform calculations and exchange information to/from the system.

The RFID part of the smart card manages procedures for registration, authentication as well as treatment. The basic components of this proposed system are:

- HIS_Healthcare information system – it ensures accessing of health information by authorised entities only.
- EHR – it is a patient's all health-related record.
- EHR_applications – this application manages the creation of a patient's record, all history of activity like scheduling proposals, patient's visits to doctors, treatment done by the doctor, other services.
- PHR – it is a combination of several online tools.
- Card for Patient-Doctor – this electronic card is an alternative for traditional health booklets used in hospitals, but it is different in form and functionality. These cards are capable of storing and transmitting health information.
- eRecipe – doctor issues an electronic prescription.

In Serbia, the architecture of electronic healthcare is a centralised system. A certificate authority manages to issue health cards and renewal of certificates. All healthcare facilities or their healthcare information system would be connected to a central database through the WAN network. Patients can access their health information from a central database by the web portal.

The server is the central database. Standard protocols such as TCP/IP, IPSec, and SSL are being used for security. The database is implemented in the SQL server. For security, new devices and systems are implemented to restrict access to certain information as per need. Different views can be created according to user rights as well as roles in the system. The Health Ministry can use all the healthcare data in the database to monitor and control drugs. The main tables are as follows:

- The "Patient" table is the central part where all data of patients is stored.
- "health_id_card" table – contains patient's data of all diseases.
- "Therapy" is a table for a patient's therapy-related data, doctor's prescription. It is to control the unauthorised usage of drugs.
- "Check" – all appointments to doctors are stored. This table can check the effectiveness of doctors. Patients ID cards have debt-related data too, which can be checked.
- An e-receipt is placed on his ID, which can be read by a pharmacist using a card reader.
- Only prescribed medicine will be visible to save sensitive data. Whatever drug is purchased by the patient will be entered.
- Any individual cannot purchase it without renewing a doctor's prescription.
- The doctor's prescription and the ID of the patient will be stored in the database.

14.6 ANONYMOUS E-PRESCRIPTIONS

From the security point of view, healthcare systems have several characteristics for consideration. The healthcare system includes a heterogeneous set of institutions and hence sometimes has conflicting goals. The whole patient's experience of medical care should be private. Hence providing confidentiality of medicine prescriptions is an important issue [3]. The pharmacist collects the information and it is often stored in databases owned by hospitals. There is no federal law for the privacy of patient's health records maintained by pharmacies. Hence the privacy of patients is compromised. There have been some examples of misuse of patient data. In medicine, a prescription is defined as "a token signed by a doctor".

There are two reasons why this is important:

(1) The prescription reveals the patient's medical history.
(2) Nowadays, insurance businesses related to healthcare are the fastest rising budget [3].

The prescription model consists of the patient, doctor, pharmacist, the entity filing the prescription, the insurer providing health benefits for enrolled patients, privacy officer, the judge responsible for legal authority, and the certification authority responsible for the medical board that grants doctors the power to issue the prescription. In this system, the first issue is access control; the second issue is to handle different resources, which can be managed under a pseudonym.

The description of the confidential prescription protocol is as follows:

- **Patient enrollment:** Firstly, every patient needs to enrol in a health insurance plan. When the patient receives this smart card, he can show his enrollment status to the doctor.
- **Patient's verification:** After enrollment in a health insurance plan, his verification process is carried out.
- **Doctor certification:** A digital certificate is issued by the Certificate Authority (CA) to doctors. This digital certificate includes details of privileges like issuing prescriptions etc. The doctor can join one or more healthcare provider organisations. After the doctor had agreed, he would be contacted by his/her provider organisation (PO). PO issues a pseudonym to the doctor.
- **Pre-approval:** The doctor connects to a digital clearinghouse to obtain pre-approval to issue a digital prescription. A form for prescription mentioning any policies will be filled.
- **Filling:** This process is as follows: (1) The patient gives his smart card to the pharmacist. (2) After reading the patient's pseudonym, the prescription is submitted one at a time to the smart card of the patient, which signs them for the pharmacist. The pharmacist forwards the digital token and collects an e-payment.

- **Anonymous profiling:** To prevent fraud, the "PBM" profile patients and "healthcare providers" profile doctors. "PBM" collect anonymous patient record together using the same pseudonym.
- **Pseudonym revocation:** Only PO would be able to open pseudonyms. It is hoped that a revocation procedure would be established.

This describes a relevant and practical system for electronic payment systems to provide privacy services to doctors and patients. It is useful, but still refinement in the security assumption is needed.

14.7 SMART-CARD-ENABLED PRIVACY-PRESERVING E-PRESCRIPTIONS SYSTEM [4]

Both patient and doctor have a security concern with this e-prescription data as other parties are involved, and some parties may use it for their benefit, like marketing etc. It has a strong proxy signature scheme that satisfies security requirements such as strong unforgettability, verifiability, identifiability. There are three types of delegation scheme – full delegation, partial delegation, and delegation by warrant. This scheme firstly provides delegation by using a strong algorithm and then a signing and verification procedure. Also, analysis of the scheme is discussed as to how all the above security parameters can be fulfilled.

As in this system smart cards play a very important role, so it becomes the target point for attack; hence, its security is a primary concern. Its memory is organised into four sections.

- Secret section: written only once, data is card manufacturers PIN, card holder's master key.
- Sensitive section: only occasional update, data are issuer's PIN, card holder's PIN.
- Working section: it can be erased and rewritten.
- Public section: no requirement for protection; anyone can read.

Patients can easily get prescriptions without any security crisis. So, this proposed system is quite practical.

14.8 PATIENT-CONTROLLED PSEUDONYM BASED EHR (PCPBEHR)

Different countries have different choices according to the needs of the community. Still, most of the popular EHR solutions argue for patient-centred as it gives total access rights to the patient. This PcPbEHR system is patient-centred, combining pseudonymisation techniques and encryption to provide an efficient mechanism for the security and privacy of the healthcare information system as shown in Figure 14.2.

If any intruder is successful in accessing the database, the patient's privacy may be compromised. Hence, to ensure strong privacy, PcPbEHR maintain two separate databases:

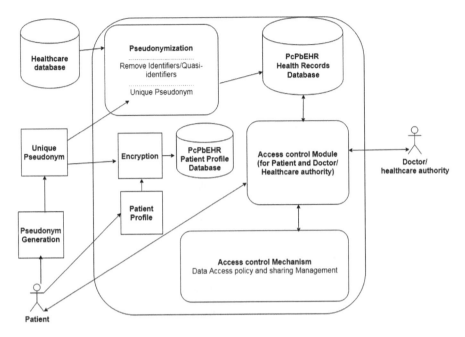

FIGURE 14.2   Architecture of PcPbEHR [20].

(1) One for identifiable information in encrypted form.
(2) Another for pseudonymised health records –the PcPbEHR health records database, which contains patient's health records after pseudonymisation.

The PcPbEHR patient profile database contains encrypted patients' profiles and encrypted patients' pseudonyms [14][20].

Before storing health records from patient/healthcare centre into the PcPbEHR health records database, the pseudonymisation module, as shown in Figure 14.3, removes all identifiers and quasi-identifiers from the patient's health record so that if an intruder gets access to the database, he/she will not be able to determine the owner of a particular health record.

Pseudonym generation is an important part of the pseudonymisation module. There are so many mechanisms that have been proposed, but it is recommended that it should be patient-centric in most cases.

All identifiable information is encrypted by a shared key, as shown in Figure 14.4. Encrypted profiles and encrypted pseudonyms are stored in a secure PcPbEHR patient profile database.

14.9   POTENTIAL OF BLOCKCHAIN AND IOT TECHNOLOGY IN HEALTHCARE

Blockchain and IoT are emerging technologies, notions and services that can provide solutions to electronic healthcare delivery, patient care and medical data management.

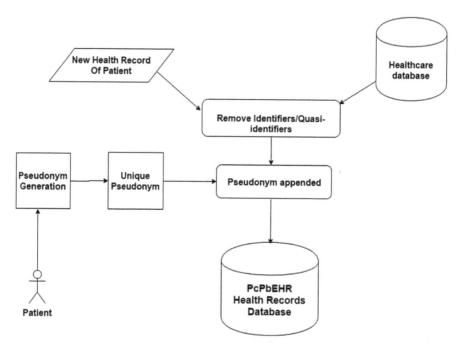

FIGURE 14.3   Pseudonymisation module [13].

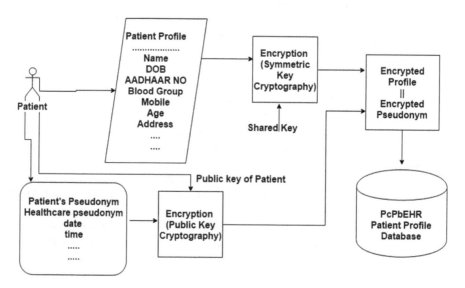

FIGURE 14.4   Encryption of patient's profile and pseudonym [20].

IoT technologies enable doctors/hospital authorities to be more watchful and retain close connection with the patients. IoT can be used for data collected from IoT devices, which can help physicians to identify the best treatment process for patients and reach the expected outcomes [21].

Recently, blockchain technology has gained immense attention due to its wide scope, ranging from cybersecurity, data management, financial services and healthcare [17][20].

Blockchain technology can be used for secure and safe data management and sharing, which is useful for effective diagnosis and treatment [17].

A variety of healthcare solutions use mobile applications, sensors or wearables. The internet is frequently used to connect, forming an IoT ecosystem. To protect health data privacy, a service-oriented architecture is required that combines all IoT solutions and a secure authentication mechanism [21].

IoT and blockchain can provide a complete solution for healthcare, facilitating the following: privacy, security, auditability, provenance, traceability, immutable data storage, etc.

14.10 CONCLUSION

Different countries make different choices according to the need of the community. Still, most popular EHR solutions argue for patient-centred as it gives total access rights to the patient. In this chapter, I have discussed several challenges of the healthcare information system and some solutions for data management, access control, privacy preservation and e-prescriptions. Most solutions advocate for the patient-centred system, a convenient, simple, privacy-preserving, secure mechanism. The availability of a patient's health information to any healthcare entity with the patient's consent is another very basic requirement. Pseudonymisation-based solutions can provide a huge opportunity for medical research on a particular disease using anonymous health data. It can provide anonymous health data that will not have any identifiable information of the patient to researchers. Hence without compromising privacy, anonymous health data will be available for researchers. Blockchain technology-based mechanisms to deal with the healthcare industry would allow users to transfer medical data safely. This would also provide users with a way to anonymously share their medical data for medical research. Blockchain technology provides a secure way to share health data and also provide improved healthcare transactions.

At present, IoT and blockchain technology have got great attention and much importance in the healthcare industry. IoT and blockchain will soon be the driving forces for healthcare information systems and numerous points of view as it is a definitive resource tracker.

Those systems that are empowered by IoT and blockchain technology have the capability of significantly decreasing the expense and the removal of current intermediates.

REFERENCES

1. Al-Hamdani, Wasim A. "Cryptography based access control in healthcare web systems," *2010 Information Security Curriculum Development Conference*, 2010. ACM.
2. Vucetic, Miljan, Uzelac, Ana, Gligoric, Nenad. "E-Health Transformation Model in Serbia: Design, Architecture and Developing," *2011 International Conference on Cyber-Enabled Distributed Computing and Knowledge Discovery*, 2011. IEEE.
3. Ateniese, Giuseppe, de Medeiros, Breno. "Anonymous e-prescriptions," *Proceedings of the 2002 ACM workshop on privacy in the Electronic Society*, 2002. ACM.
4. Yang, Yanjiang, et al. "A smart-card-enabled privacy preserving E-prescription system," *IEEE Transactions on Information Technology in Biomedicine*, 8(1), 2004, 47–58.
5. Slamanig, Daniel, Stingl, Christian. "Privacy aspects of e-health," *2008 Third International Conference on Availability, Reliability and Security*, 2008. IEEE.
6. Peterson, Robert. "Encryption system for allowing immediate universal access to medical records while maintaining complete patient control over privacy," US Patent Application No. 09/973,796.
7. Thielscher, Christian, et al. "Patent: Data processing system for patient data," *Int. Patent, WO* 3.034294, 2005, A2.
8. Pommerening, Klaus, Reng, Michael. "Secondary use of the EHR via pseudonymisation," *Studies in health technology and informatics*, 2004, 441–446.
9. Røstad, Lillian. "Access Control in Healthcare Applications," *Access Control in Healthcare Information Systems*, 2008, 37.
10. Ni, Qun, et al. "Privacy-aware role-based access control," *ACM Transactions on Information and System Security (TISSEC)*, 13(3), 2010, 24.
11. Rai, Bipin Kumar, et al. "Security and Privacy Issues in Healthcare Information System," *International Journal of Emerging Trends & Technology in Computer Science (IJETTCS)*, 3(6), 2014.
12. Rai, Bipin Kumar, et al. "Pseudonymization Techniques for Providing Privacy and Security in EHR," in *International Journal of Emerging Trends & Technology in Computer Science (IJETTCS)*, 5(4), 2016.
13. Rai, Bipin Kumar, et al. "Patient controlled Pseudonym-based mechanism suitable for privacy and security of Electronic Health Record," *International Journal of Research in Engineering, IT and Social Sciences*, 588, (7.2), 2017.
14. Rai, Bipin Kumar, et al. "Prototype Implementation of Patient controlled Pseudonym-based mechanism for Electronic Health Record (PcPbEHR)," *International Journal of Research in Engineering, IT and Social Sciences*, 588: 7(7), 2017.
15. Dekker, Mari Antonius Cornelis, Etalle, Sandro. "Audit-based access control for electronic health records," *Electronic Notes in Theoretical Computer Science*, 168, 2007, 221–236.
16. Kulkarni, Devdatta, Tripathi, Anand. "Context-aware role-based access control in pervasive computing systems," *Proceedings of the 13th ACM symposium on Access control models and technologies*, 2008. ACM.
17. Ananth, C., Karthikeyan, M., Mohananthini, N. "A secured healthcare system using private blockchain technology," *J. Eng. Technol*, 6, 2018, 42–54.
18. Aziz, H. A., Guled, A. "Cloud computing and healthcare services," 2016.
19. http://docs.oasis-open.org/xacml/3.0/xacml-3.0-core-spec-cs-01-en.pdf.
20. Rai, Bipin Kumar, *Pseudonymisation Based Mechanism for Security & Privacy of Healthcare*, 2020, LAMBERT Academic Publishing.
21. Garcia, Nuno M., Pires, Ivan Miguel, Goleva, Rossitza, "IoT Technologies for HealthCare," in *6th EAI International Conference, HealthyIoT 2019*, December 4–6, 2019, DOI:10.1007/978-3-030-42029-1.

Index

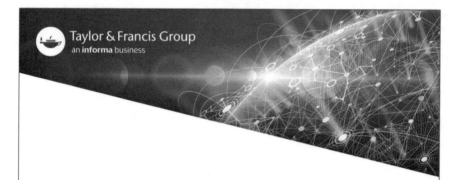